TRAIL OF THE SPIRIT

TRAIL OF THE SPIRIT

The Mysteries of
Medicine Power Revealed

George Blondin

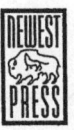

Copyright © George Blondin 2006

All rights reserved. The use of any part of this publication reproduced, transmitted in any form or by any means, electronic, mechanical, recording or otherwise, or stored in a retrieval system, without the prior consent of the publisher is an infringement of the copyright law. In the case of photocopying or other reprographic copying of the material, a license must be obtained from Access Copyright before proceeding.

Library and Archives Canada Cataloguing in Publication
Blondin, George, 1922-
Trail of the spirit : the mysteries of medicine power revealed / George Blondin.

ISBN-13: 978-1-897126-08-0 (pbk.)
ISBN-10: 1-897126-08-5 (pbk.)

1. Tinne Indians--Medicine. 2. Tinne Indians--Folklore. I. Title.

E99.T56T73 2006   615.8'808997   C2006-905264-6

Editor for the Board: Richard Van Camp
Cover and interior design: Katherine Melnyk
Cover image: T. Macintosh/NWT Archive—
"Spirit of the drum Eddie Weyallon & students, Rae sunrise, 1992."
Author Photo: Rene Fumoleau
Illustrations by: Era Novak and Liora Salter

NeWest Press acknowledges the support of the Canada Council for the Arts, the Alberta Foundation for the Arts, and the Edmonton Arts Council for our publishing program. We also acknowledge the financial support of the Government of Canada through the Book Publishing Industry Development Program (BPIDP).

NeWest Press
201–8540–109 Street
Edmonton, Alberta T6G 1E6
(780) 432-9427
www.newestpress.com

NeWest Press is committed to protecting the environment and to the responsible use of natural resources. This book is printed on 100% recycled, ancient-forest friendly paper.

3 4 5 23 22 21

PRINTED AND BOUND IN CANADA

Table of Contents

Acknowledgements ix
Forward by Richard Van Camp 1
Note from Ted Blondin 5
Introduction 7
Chapter 1: Believing in Medicine Power 14
       2: First-Class Medicine Power 16
       3: What is a Spirit? 19
       4: Eligibility for Medicine Power 22
       5: Yamoria 23
       6: Yamagah, Brother of Yamoria 28
       7: Yamagah: the Story Continues 35
       8: Medicine-Power Law 38
       9: The Story of Edwar 45
       10: The Story of Kenny 49
       11: Space and the Planets 55
       12: Spirits and the Gift of Medicine Power 59
       13: The Story of Paul Blondin 61
       14: The Story of Bahwar and Yendee 67
       15: The Story of Ehdah 80
       16: Lost! 85
       17: Dene Prayer 88
       18: The Way of Prophets and Miracles 90
       19: The Challenges of Living with Medicine Power 92
       20: Medicine Power for Eagle 97
       21: The Prophecies of Ehtseo Ayah 99
       22: The Story of Teleway 100
       23: Medicine Power for the Wind 107
       24: Monster Medicine Power 109
       25: Monster Medicine Power II 113

26: Comparing Medicine Power 116
27: A Powerful Medicine Person as Leader. 119
28: War Using Medicine Power 120
29: Medicine Power and Hand Games 127
30: The Story of Bechachy. 133
31: The Story of Gotaregai 140
32: The Story of Edzo. 144
33: The Rabbitskin People. 153
34: The Rabbitskin and Chipewyan Nations at War 156
35: The Story of Sahlie 158
36: The Baby Survives! 164
37: The Story of Batimie 166
38: The Story of Adam 169
39: The Story of Tosoih Taha 171
40: The Sick Woman is Cured! 173
41: How Medicine Power Stopped Violence in a Family . . . 175
42: The Leader of the Caribou 176
43: Whiskey Jack Medicine 178
44: The Year of Two Winters 179
Conclusion. 181
Author Biography 182

Acknowledgements

THE PREPARATION TO HAVE THIS BOOK WRITTEN, EDITED, AND PUBLISHED was no easy task. I would like to thank the following people for their assistance to get us to this point. I would like to thank Rita Chretien for editing my father's notes and managing to produce the first manuscript. I would like to thank Rudy Wiebe for convincing the NeWest Press Board to publish this book. I want to thank Liora Salter for responding so quickly in the short period of time and drawing the pictures in this book. I would also like to thank the staff of NeWest Press for spending the many hours communicating long distance in organizing various tasks that had to get done to meet our deadlines. I want to also thank Richard Van Camp for doing the final editing and working with NeWest and myself to finalize this book. Last but not least, I want to thank the people of the North for the overwhelming support provided to my father, not only for this book, but for all the other initiatives he was involved in. Read these stories to your children and help keep the Dene culture alive. Enjoy!

Ted Blondin

Foreword by Richard Van Camp

THE FIRST TIME I EVER MET GEORGE BLONDIN WAS IN 1990. I WAS IN Yellowknife studying Native Management Studies at Aurora College. At that time, I was considering living my life as a land claims negotiator for my people, the Dogribs of the Treaty 11 area. George was promoting his first book, *When the World was New*. In the hour or so George spoke with us about his book and did a reading, he transported me to an incredible time in Dene history where Yamoria made the land safe for us all. He also spoke about medicine, which surprised me because most Dene Elders do not speak so openly about it. And for that I was grateful because he made me proud of my inheritance as a member of the Dene Nation. When I met George Blondin, I was humbled because I was shaking hands with someone who has dedicated his life to documenting the stories, beliefs, and philosophies of the Dene people of the Northwest Territories, and he has inspired me over the years to blaze my own trail with my writing.

In *Trail of the Spirit*, George documents with great passion the Dene beliefs behind medicine power, and he brings to life with cinematic prowess the lives of Dene heroes like Paul Blondin, Kenny, Edwar, Bahwar, Yendee, Ehdah, Akaitcho, Edzo, and several more. As well, he illuminates the relationship of Yamoria and his brother, Yamagah, and George also shares the laws that Yamoria put forth for the Dene of Denendeh to live by.

These stories are such great medicine for all who read them, and what a testament to the power of oral history this is as it has taken George thirteen years to write this book. Each time I read these stories, I feel that George makes the transition from oral history to literature so seamlessly you're not even aware he does it—until days later when you realize that you can see and feel exactly what it is he has told you. Take, for instance, the friendship George captures between Kenny and Paul

Blondin in Chapter 12. I ache for the ability to capture that in my own writing: the friendship between two men. George is sharing this story but making it his own with his medicine as a storyteller to make it a story we can all relate to, regardless of where we come from. We understand that these two are brothers for life. Chapter 33 is writing at its finest: I won't give it away, but the language and descriptions in that chapter take my breath away just thinking about what George has captured.

George also shares three very powerful stories of peace in this collection, and for that I give thanks, because this is the first time I've ever read the story of how the Dogribs and the Chipewyan, and the Rabbitskin people and the Chipewyan, made peace after decades of out-butchering each other. As well, George shares a humorous piece about how two fierce enemies, Yamagah and Eyonee Cho, not only made peace, they chose to live together and to become friends after years of battling. I say the story is humorous because their final battle is so feeble I chuckle every time I read it. I think in these times of international conflict, we have a lot to learn from these stories. The great warriors, Edzo and Akaitcho, made peace after admitting that if the peace did not begin between leaders that the wars between their people would never end. The same with Eyonee Cho and Yamagah: they know they are evenly matched, and it is Yamagah who invites Eyonee Cho to live with him and his people after their worst battle. Again, both men have lost their closest loved ones and learn to live together as friends—despite that last pitiful fistfight between them when they are ancient and mumblers!

Another great thing George does in this book is that he shares the prophecies and miracles of Ehtseo Ayah of Déline and Teleway from the Colville Lake area, and he shares stories that have not been available in the written word before.

And, once again, I am humbled and inspired by George Blondin as an author and lover of great Aboriginal literature.

My wish for you is to sit back, relax, read these stories, and enjoy them, for they've been gathered by one of our finest listeners and storytellers.

Then pass on the teachings and stories gathered here, for they've been gathered by a generous heart, and someone who wants the stories of the Dene people to survive forever. . . .

Mahsi cho!

Richard Van Camp
Vancouver, BC, 2006

Note from Ted Blondin

As long as I can remember, my father has been telling stories to whoever will listen. I didn't understand then that he was doing this—not because he was good at it, but because it was his destiny and responsibility to pass these very important stories to future generations. It was very important to my father to explain and maintain a very important part of our culture, as Dene People—the real custodians of our lands—to continue our stability and responsibility to our land, our people and our future.

In an age of information, my father found it difficult to maintain this responsibility along with the younger generation due to the added influence of TV, Nintendo games, and the Internet, as opposed to stories

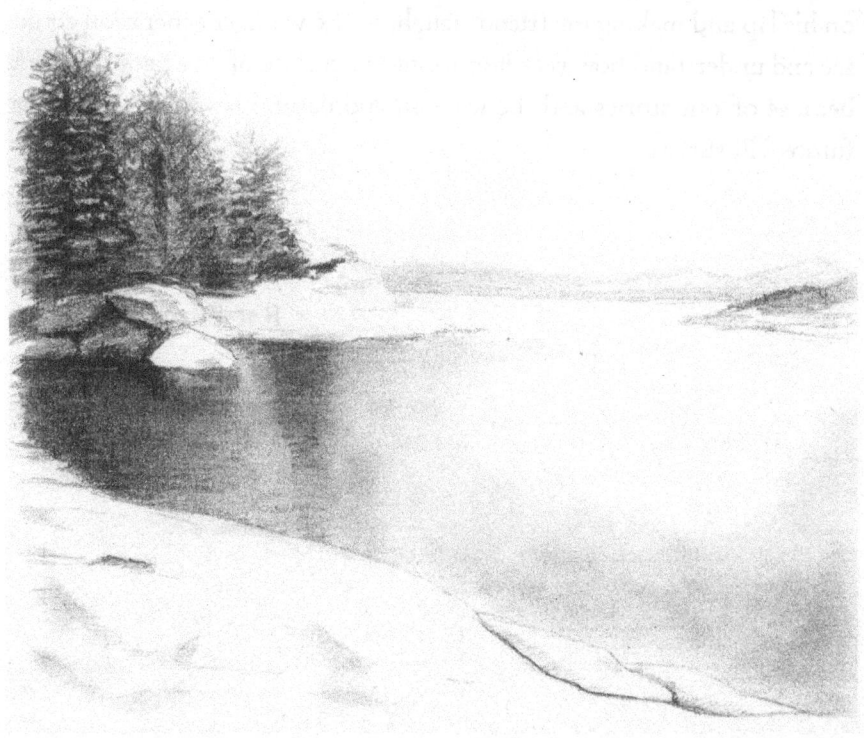

around the campfires during his younger days. To keep these important stories of his people alive, he broke some important rules: not to talk about sacred issues, such as "medicine power." He wrote his first book, *When The World Was New* by candlelight in his cabin while trapping at Megil Bay on the north shore of Great Bear Lake. His second book, *Yamoria: The Lawmaker*, was about stories that were told by elders throughout the North of the most powerful medicine man who made new laws between animals and humans that maintained a close interaction for the survival of both groups to this day.

There are many stories such as these published by different Aboriginal groups across Canada, but none of these books ever went into great detail as to what this special phenomenon was to make the general public know what it was! My father goes into great detail as to how to explain what "medicine power" is and defines it.

I hope you enjoy these stories as I have: when I was very young, sitting on his lap and making my friends laugh, so the younger generation could see and understand how very important the culture of our people is and, because of our stories and the wisdom and natural laws they carry, our future will survive.

Ted Blondin
A Very Proud Son
Rae-Edzo, NWT, 2006

Introduction

I was born north of Great Bear Lake in the Barren lands, just like the Inuit. The year was 1923. This makes me eighty-three years of age.

In the period of that time, the area was very isolated in terms of who governed Canada. There was no law, no RCMP, no priest, and no government. The Dene would go to a small store at Fort Norman, NWT, which is three hundred miles away from where I was born. They used dog teams in the winter and canoes in the summer to get there.

They told me when I was born that I was the first boy born in the family; therefore, we have in our culture a practice to take the baby to a man with medicine powers to hold the baby and to try to push medicine powers inside the baby. Sometimes the baby boy received medicine power like that. Not only that, but some strong medicine-power people could predict how long the baby would live. My mom and dad told me later, "We tried everything for you to be a medicine-power person, but we failed. You must be a bad man, but some of these people say you would live a long life." This was true, and my parents were happy about it.

As I grew to four or six years old, I had two grandfathers. They were small-time medicine-power people. I spent a lot of the time with them, yet I never received medicine power. I must be bad. When I reached seven years old, my parents sent me to a mission school run by the church and the nuns. I stayed four years in that school. I got to grade three in school and I returned to my parents.

In 1930, in the Great Bear Lake area, when I stayed in school, they forbid me to talk Indian. Therefore, I spoke only broken English. But when I got back to my parents, they forbid me to talk English.

For the next fifteen years, I stayed in the bush with my parents. I forgot that when I went to school I could not talk English. I just stayed in the bush and did what I was supposed to do. In the summer you fish with fishnets. You make a lot of dry fish for next winter. You hunt moose, shoot ducks, and snare rabbits. That is our summer job. In the winter you trap. You trap furs for the Hudson's Bay Company. At the store, you get what you need. As I think about life, at that time there was no communication with the outside world; therefore, you don't know what is going on. It's because you don't talk English. You don't read or write. So you don't know what goes on. We didn't know that World War II was on, so after fifteen years in the bush it was 1945. I got married and had three kids of my own. I became aware that my kids needed to go to school, but there was no school in the country. In Yellowknife there was a school. I decided to go to Yellowknife. It was about eight hundred miles away. I loaded my wife and kids on my toboggan and travelled to Yellowknife. It took me one and a half months to get there, but I started to live there.

I found a job in the mine. I worked there for eleven years. It was a hard life. My wife Julia died during that eleven years. My kids grew up. All of them went to school, some time around 1960. I was all alone. My kids received their education and began to take care of themselves. I decided to go back in the bush to trap and hunt.

Some time later, I went back to Yellowknife again, and there was a group of Dene people who had established an organization to settle land claims with the government. They invited me to work with them. I agreed. It was just like going to school again. In no time I started to learn a lot about politics and how the government governed Canada. Also, I learned that the government does not treat Indians fairly.

In ten years of work there, I became the vice president of that organization. I became a very political person. I learned a lot about the general movement of the problems of the Indian people. The lifestyle of the Dene started to change because education was there in the north. Some Dene were not interested in hunting and trapping. I, myself, became not interested in bush life anymore, so, during that period, I started changing my lifestyle. That is when I got real interested in my own Dene people and how they survived in the past. I wrote a lot about them for local papers in Yellowknife. Soon, I was interested in writing a book about my own people and how they survived. I wrote two good books in two years. It was interesting. It's because I grew up among a lot of Indian storytellers. The Indians are wonderful storytellers. I learned a lot from them. They go back in time roughly eighty thousand years and tell stories of giant animals like dinosaurs and Eagles, a lot of different types of giant animals and birds. They talk like their stories happened yesterday. All Indians are wonderful storytellers. They also talk about medicine power. That's where I learned a lot, so writing two books was no problem. So about thirteen years ago I decided to write my last book. I thought I could define medicine power and that readers would be interested in how, in the past, great medicine-power people did great action that was hard to believe because medicine power is very broad. Even Indian storytellers talk a lot about it. It's still not good enough to cover the definition of medicine power, but, in my thinking, I thought a book of that kind would be very interesting to everybody.

This book is my attempt at doing something no one else has ever done: to define medicine power. The period in time that this work discusses is the past two hundred years, although medicine power has existed since time began. I will bring to life medicine power for you in the way of the Dene storyteller, by describing real events in Dene history. It is my hope that through this journey a better understanding and a clear explanation of medicine power will be achieved. Here you will find a collection of stories and examples of Dene individuals who lived throughout history and how they used medicine power for both good and destruction.

In the beginning, when the world was new, the two-legged nation walked upon Mother Earth. For a long time this nation acted more like animals than the human beings we know of today. They were wild. Then something very important happened. Yamoria brought Dene law to the people.

Yamoria was a very powerful medicine man and prophet. He was a true holy man who taught the Dene how to live a sacred life. He travelled all over the land speaking to groups of people wherever he went. His life's mission was to transform the whole nation into a community of loving people who worked in harmony with each other for the good of all. Yamoria also taught the people how to live with medicine power.

Medicine power—what is it? "It's a mystery," they say. "Where did the power come from in the first place?" they ask. It is a topic that is hard to understand and even more difficult to explain because it is a spirit. The Elders teach that medicine power is a gift from the Creator, when, really, it is just a loan. When there is no need for it, it will be gone. I worry that medicine power is being extinguished today.

In the beginning, when the world was new, animals, fish, and birds lived on Mother Earth, but human beings did not. It was like this for a very long time. Still, the creatures that lived on Mother Earth at that time had medicine power.

All Aboriginal people, in ancient times, were familiar with medicine power because their lives depended on it. It didn't matter whether someone was a medicine person or not; he or she still believed in and relied on medicine power. Even if someone did not possess their own powers, they got help from those who did. This is true of Aboriginal people all over Mother Earth.

Dene people have always believed in God, the Creator of all things. When the missionaries arrived in this country, they told our people that medicine power came from the devil and they did not want us using it or even believing in it.

Ayah, the great Dene prophet from Déline, Northwest Territories, who passed away in 1940, taught a great deal about the Creator. He told the people that the missionaries were wrong. He reassured, "The Devil has made nothing. The Creator has made everything. Medicine power is a gift from the Creator to the Dene because we need it so badly to survive. But it is only on loan from the Creator and it cannot stay with us forever. Someday, in the future, when we no longer need it, it will disappear as if the Creator has taken it back."

We ask, "How is this strong, invisible, medicine-power spirit given to each individual all over Mother Earth and who does the giving?" Obviously, nothing is impossible for the Creator of all things. We do believe that the Creator, God, is everywhere. When a poor man prays with his whole heart, alone in his tent in the bush, the Creator will come to him and be right beside him, listening and ready to help. For the billions of people on Mother Earth, the Creator, God, listens to each one and helps them.

It is believed that one has to be very good, almost holy, to receive medicine power. If a person is not pure of heart they will not receive medicine power. The Creator, who knows and sees all, can determine whether or not someone will have the qualities necessary to use medicine power. The Creator distributes medicine power in a variety of ways; the most powerful of medicine people receive their gifts before they are born. The gift of medicine power is given to the individual to help them with their life on earth and so that they can help their people. It is considered great fortune to receive medicine power in this way. Others work very hard in hopes that they will earn medicine power someday.

The most powerful medicine is the medicine given to a lucky individual before he is born. His spirit would receive the gift as the strongest medicine power because it came directly from the Creator. There is no equal to this medicine power. This is genuine medicine power and the individual has to look after it all his life, and he can do anything he likes because he owns the power he received.

A second way to receive medicine power is at the time of your birth. There is still not much information on this topic, since the baby is too small, but the medicine power is still genuine power. In time, the baby would get a vision of medicine power. Possibly, a man would try to teach the baby as he or she grew until the baby would really know how to handle the medicine power properly. The baby would become an adult and handle the medicine power by him or herself.

The third way to receive medicine power is for it to be passed to you from someone else. For example, sometimes parents or grandparents give some or all of their medicine power to their children just before they leave the physical world and return to the spirit world, where they no longer need it. This is the least desirable way to receive medicine power because it is not as strong as when you receive it before you are born. It does not work well because it does not come from the Creator. Some Elder had claimed he had given part of his medicine power to his son. This type of medicine, which a lot of people get involved in, is bad because people can make a lot of mistakes. They get into trouble. Sadly, people die because of this. A lot of people die young before their time. A lot of Elders don't like this type of movement because it is too much trouble and is very dangerous.

The strongest of medicine people usually have a great vision that guides them throughout their life. Their vision explains many things to them, such as how to use their medicine power. Although the teaching within the vision is very deep and extensive, it happens in an instant.

I have had the privilege of listening to four different people explain to me how they received medicine power before they were born. One man said, "I have medicine power for everything on earth: the wind, clouds, air, sun, moon, planets, the space, fog, and water. Also, I have power for all the creatures that walk and crawl upon the earth, and those that fly in the sky. I have medicine power for things that grow and even the minds of animals and human beings."

Another way of working with medicine power is to become a partner with the spirit of an animal. When this happens, the medicine person speaks the same language as the spirit animal. They work as a team. However, this could even happen with other things such as rocks. We know from the teachings of the prophets that all things have a spirit.

Medicine power comes in many forms. It is possible to work with the medicine-power spirit of the wind or the moon and many, many other things. When a medicine power, such as the wind, works with a medicine person, it takes a certain form that assists them to communicate. It could even be similar to a human form. The medicine-power spirit may say, "I am the wind. If you want something done, I could help you."

This is just the beginning of explaining medicine power.

1: Believing in Medicine Power

DENE PEOPLE BELIEVE THAT THE CREATOR, GOD, CREATED EVERYTHING on this earth. Why some things are visible to us and other things are not, such as air or the spirit world, is a great mystery. Even Christianity teaches that it is valuable to believe, even in things you cannot see.

Remember the story in the Bible when Jesus died on the cross? His spirit appeared to his disciples, all but one: Thomas, who was not there at the time. Later, when Thomas was told that Jesus had appeared to the other disciples, he could not believe it. He said, "I will only believe it if I see it with my own eyes." Then Jesus appeared to him and showed him his wounded hands and feet. Thomas knelt down and said, "My God, it's you." Jesus replied, "Thomas, you see and now you believe. Blessed are those who do not see but still believe."

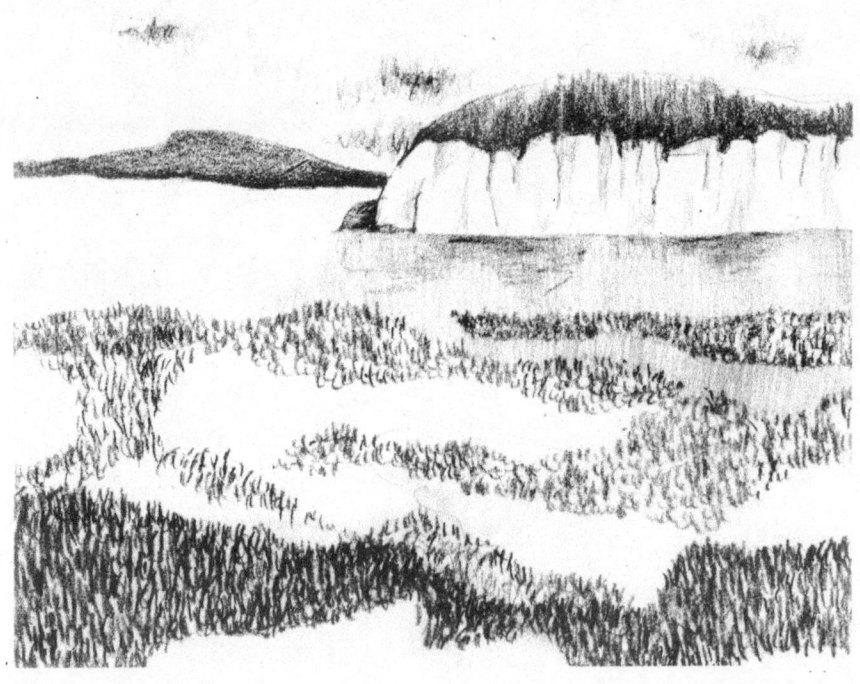

It is the same with medicine power. Although the person who does not possess medicine power may not be able to see or hear the medicine-power spirits, they still do exist. It's alright if you find this hard to understand. It will become clearer as we go along.

The Bible says there are some things that we will only really understand when we go to heaven. This is true of many things on this earth. Why do millions of people die in the great wars? Or why do individuals have to endure so much suffering when they lose their young wives, husbands, or children? We can be comforted that the mysteries of life shall all be revealed when we return to the spirit world.

We also must trust that the Creator has a plan for everything here on Mother Earth, even when we can't understand it. It is not helpful to become angry with the Creator because he is the greatest spirit that exists. Instead, we pray to the Creator.

The Bible says that people have a soul. It also says that your spirit separates from your body when you die. I do not know the difference between the spirit and the soul. I believe that we each have only one spirit. Medicine power is also a spirit.

Medicine people have the ability to communicate with your spirit. They tell us that we each have a spirit that is attached to our physical bodies. In fact, you cannot survive without your spirit. How do they know this? Medicine people can see it. When a medicine person is asked to help someone who is sick, often the first thing they do is check to see if the patient still has his or her spirit. If it is gone, they know the person will not live much longer.

Long ago, medicine people were known to steal a person's spirit and cause them to die.

2: First-Class Medicine Power

When the world was new, it was necessary to know not only who a medicine person was but also who was a very strong medicine person and could be depended on. Dene people truly were dependant upon medicine power to survive and, therefore, it was a crucial aspect of life. Still, because medicine power is a spirit, most medicine people would not talk about their medicine power. Fortunately for us, some medicine people did talk about their medicine power and that is how we've learned what we know about medicine power today.

This story is about a man from Fort Norman, NWT, who was an unusual medicine man. He owned only one medicine power and it was a strange power. There was no way for him to help others with this medicine power. Yet, he was a happy person, always joking and worry free. He had medicine power for his skin.

Each spring when the weather began to get warm, his skin would turn real dark and scaly. When the scales peeled off, he looked miserable and ugly. The people knew this was from his medicine power and would laugh at him. Women would tell him, "You look ugly! Why don't you get rid of that stupid medicine power? You suffer too much."

But he'd just answer, "I can't! It's my medicine power and, besides, it will help me to live a long life." Then he'd laugh.

That man lived to one hundred years old. He was poor all his life. He was not a successful hunter, trapper, or fisherman because he did not have medicine power for these things. He did not help his people to survive with his medicine power.

Then there's Edwar of Aklavik who you will read about in Chapter 10. He was just the opposite. Edwar had too much medicine power. He had so many different items of power that it would take forever to name them all. To give the title "medicine man" to both of these men seems inadequate. We do not have language to describe different kinds of medicine people, but, as you can see in this story, they can be very different. Dene people only have a name to describe a medicine person who is very powerful and can overpower other medicine people. That name is *Beh Bah Teh*. But, I think we should create names to identify different types of medicine people too.

I suggest that we call medicine people who have received their medicine power before they were born "first-class medicine-power people," and medicine people who received their medicine power after they were born, "second-class medicine-power people." Then, medicine people who were passed their medicine power from their grandfather or relations could be called "third-class medicine-power people."

People who receive their medicine power sometimes have bought their medicine power, which doesn't actually work very well. Perhaps it's because they have not received the power directly from the Creator. It's also possible that the spirit of the medicine power is not entirely committed to this person and, therefore, the third-class medicine person isn't in control of the medicine power. Third-class medicine power is not reliable. Sometimes it works; sometimes it does not.

Those of us who are not medicine people cannot distinguish between the different kinds of medicine people. Word spreads quickly when someone is identified as a medicine person and, soon afterward, people approach the medicine person for help, even though they do not know what kind of powers the person possesses.

If a third-class medicine person is arrogant, he may be tempted to pretend that he has powers that he does not. He may even try to fake his powers to fool people. Medicine-power spirits are very powerful and not to be played with. A third-class medicine person will eventually end up in trouble if he does this.

For example, the right protocol for a medicine person to receive help from the spirit of the medicine power is for him or her to approach the spirit first just to communicate about the ceremony. This way they are in agreement about how to proceed. But, if the medicine person is acting out of pride and arrogance, he or she may not follow this protocol. This is a way to die young and quick. They say many young third-class medicine people have lost their lives this way. Medicine power is nothing to play with!

All kinds of medicine powers are genuine. Still, it's useful to be able to distinguish between the three different kinds of medicine power. First-class medicine power is much stronger than second-class medicine power because it is given directly from the Creator before you are born into this physical world. Second-class medicine power is received after you are born, through visions and a messenger from the Creator. Third-class medicine power is not as strong as second-class medicine power because it is passed from one person to another.

First-class medicine power is capable of knowing all the things that have happened in the past, are happening in the present, and will happen in the future. This medicine power also has knowledge of all things on Mother Earth and beyond. A medicine person who has first-class medicine power would have complete knowledge of medicine power and how it works and has access to this infinite knowledge.

All medicine-power people are visited daily from a spirit helper who teaches them the workings of medicine power. However, high-class medicine-power people can communicate with all levels of medicine power: high, middle, and low. But low- or middle-class medicine-power people cannot communicate with higher levels of medicine power than what they possess. For example, a low-class medicine man cannot communicate with a high-class medicine power.

Only a high-class medicine-power person, which is truly very rare, could make a deal with a high-class medicine-power spirit. The medicine power respects the medicine-power person and this is essential or the medicine power would likely just ignore their requests. Truly, the medicine person needs assistance to help heal someone. This is when they ask for help from the very high-class medicine power, as they don't have any trouble communicating with the spirit of the medicine power.

The Creator gives out medicine power to individuals. The Creator knows everything, including what kind of persons those individuals will be, even before they are born. The spirit of that individual is the one who receives the medicine power for life. So if you wonder how a person can receive medicine power before they were born, it's actually the spirit of the individual who receives the medicine power. Then the person is born and becomes a medicine person at birth.

3: What is a Spirit?

DENE STORYTELLERS HAVE MANY STORIES ABOUT THINGS THAT HAPPEN when you die. They say that at the time of your death your spirit departs from your body and travels to the spirit world. There it can be born into this physical world again. It is a circle. In fact, because Dene storytellers have so much to say about the spirit, we have a special word to describe the spirit once it has left the physical body. It is *Incha Dene*.

Dene people believe that the spirit is attached to your body. It stays inside your body and this is the power that makes you live. If your spirit leaves your physical body for any reason, your body will die soon afterward. Of course, only your physical body dies, because your spirit is eternal. It can never die. Every person on Mother Earth has a spirit of his or her own.

When a medicine person has medicine for spirit, it means he or she can go to the spirit world and look around. He or she actually becomes a spirit and traces the trail a spirit has taken. They can then talk to the spirit and return to the physical world. A medicine person who sees that someone's spirit has left their body knows that they will die soon, unless the spirit can be returned to the body somehow.

BEH GAHLEY (TRAIL OF THE SPIRIT)

Some medicine people have a special ability. They can explore the journey of your life. This is called *Beh Gahley*, or the "Trail of the Spirit." It is a trail that reaches both back into your past to the time of your birth and into your future to the time of your death. A medicine person who looks at your *Beh Gahley*, or trail of your spirit, could tell you how long you will live. Of course, not all medicine people have this unique ability. Only those who were gifted with medicine power for *Beh Gahley* will be able to do this. Here is a story that will illustrate this teaching.

One day a family arrived at a large camp. They were very distressed and asked to see a medicine person. Their ten-year-old daughter was very sick and they were afraid that she would die. They were taken to a well-known medicine man who immediately asked for the girl, "Bring the girl to me. I've been expecting you." Straight away, he checked the girl's spirit and sadly found that it was gone. "I will have to perform a ceremony to see *Beh Gahley*," he said.

The medicine man reviewed the young girl's life and uncovered the source of her illness. The family had been travelling along the lakeshore where the snow had drifted in great mounds. To make camp and set up their tent, they cut the brush on top of the snowdrift. At that point the girl was healthy. She was outside playing with a small sled. Up the snow hill she would pull the sled. Then down the hill she flew right atop the drifted snow. She played late into the night, yelling and making a racket and having great fun.

However, unbeknownst to the family, they had mistakenly pitched their tent right where an old and powerful medicine woman had died. The young girl had been sliding and playing right above where the old woman had been buried. For some reason, the spirit of the medicine woman was still tied to this place where she had died and she did not appreciate the noise of the girl's play. Selfishly, the old woman spirit stole the girl's spirit. She wanted to keep the girl's spirit with her for company, even though she knew that the girl would die.

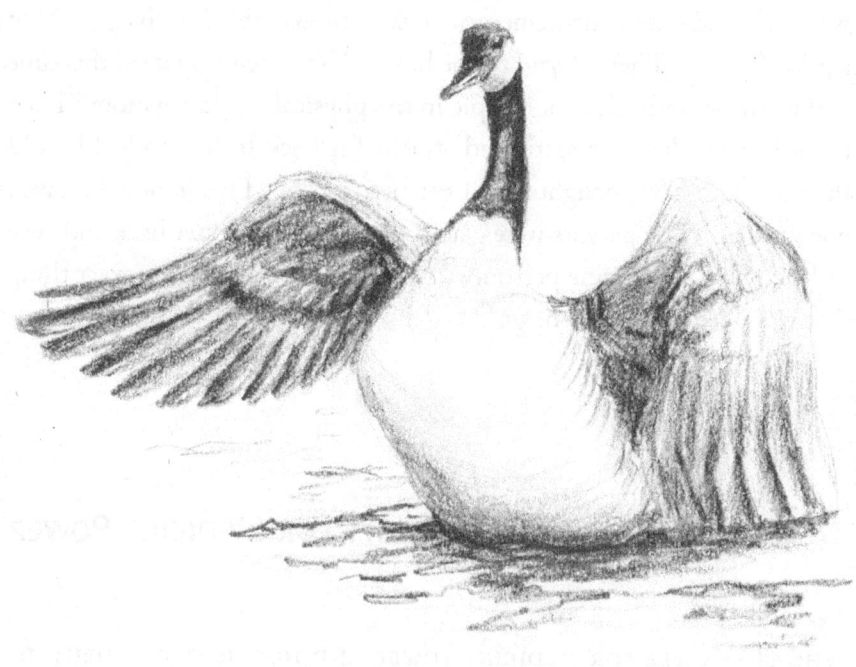

The medicine man who performed the *Beh Gahley* ceremony had many gifts. He also had medicine power similar to the old medicine woman, who was now in the spirit world. This meant he could easily talk to the old woman. "What have you done, old woman? I see the girl's spirit that you are carrying there. You will have to give it to me now."

"No!" she refused, "I am so lonesome. I will keep the girl's spirit with me." The medicine man continued to try to persuade her: "I'm sorry you are so lonely, but it does not belong to you. This spirit belongs to the girl, and if you keep it she will die. Her parents will suffer too much. Besides, what you have done is not right. Now give it to me."

Still the old woman refused. The medicine man tried a different tactic. "Then I will have to kill you," he said. The old woman laughed, "How can you kill me? I already died once and I can't die again!"

"Yes you can. And I will have to kill you because you are interfering with people in the physical world," he said. With that, he struck the old woman's head with a medicine-power axe. She crumbled to the ground in a pile of bones. Then he said to the bones, "You are really dead this time and won't be bothering the people in the physical world anymore." Then he picked up the girl's spirit and attached it back to her body. He told the parents, "Your daughter will get better now." This is how he saved one girl's life. The parents were glad to have their daughter back and very lucky to find a medicine person with medicine power for the exact thing that was needed to save the girl.

4: Eligibility for Medicine Power

Who is eligible for medicine power and how is it distributed? Medicine power comes to individuals in various ways. Sometimes a messenger, who is working for the Creator, brings the powerful gifts. Messengers come in many forms, such as an animal spirit, or an old man or woman. They are different for each person who receives medicine power and, as I've said before, may present himself, or herself, to the medicine person before or after they are born into this physical world.

I have heard of messengers coming in the form of a moose, caribou, or bear. The caribou spirit communicates with the medicine person and may say something like, "I am here representing the caribou. I give to you medicine power from my nation so that we can work together to help all the nations on Mother Earth."

It is said that one has to be a "good person" to receive medicine power.

5: YAMORIA

AT ONE TIME, THERE WAS A FAMILY THAT LIVED NEAR A FISH LAKE. THE elderly man and his wife had a daughter who was a young woman. Each day, the old man visited his fishnets and rabbit snares. His daughter had her own rabbit snares and checked them everyday, as well.

One evening, the daughter noticed a small tree moving. As she studied it she became convinced that something strange was happening. The wind was not blowing and the nearby bushes and trees were not moving—only this one small tree. Back and forth, back and forth; it seemed the tree had a rhythm to it.

When she returned to her parents that night, she described what she had seen. They had seen many unusual things in their lives and thought little of it. They counseled her, "When you go back to your rabbit snares tomorrow, check the tree again. If it moves, kneel in front of it and tell it that you are there to listen to anything it has to say to you."

The next day she was anxious to visit that small tree and see if it had something to tell her. She hurried to the same spot to find the tree swaying back and forth as it had the day before. She knelt down as her parents had instructed her, but, before she could say a word, the tree fell to the ground. As she examined the exposed roots, she noticed the dirt moving. Then she heard a baby cry. She looked under the roots and saw two babies. She gently picked each one up and placed them inside her garment, next to her skin.

She hurried back to camp and to her parents: "Mom! Dad! I found two babies! I found two babies!" The parents raised these two boys as their own and they grew up to be two very powerful and famous medicine men: Yamoria and Yamagah.

Yamoria and his brother were very happy growing up with their adopted parents. They loved them very much. The parents had great respect for the boys while they were growing up. The parents recognized the boys were special people who came from Mother Earth. The parents were aware of the boys' great medicine-power spirits who taught the boys everything. The parents also knew how to handle and work with medicine power and were careful in raising the boys properly for their lives ahead.

Yamoria had vision power, an element of medicine power that informed Yamoria about the existence of all matters in the universe since the beginning of time. This is how Yamoria acquired information about things. All he needed to do was say some words in medicine-power language, and that particular medicine power responded to his command.

Yamoria is considered "The Great Lawmaker," and he brought a way of life to the Dene that is based on these laws. They changed the way we lived and worked with each other.

Yamoria and Yamagah discussed the lifestyle of the people. They did this by flying around together with their spirits and studying what the people were doing. When the world was new, there were all kinds of people living together and medicine people were everywhere.

They say that people did not act as human beings. Instead, they behaved more like wild animals fighting one another. Another problem was that the medicine people used their medicine power to hurt one another. They abused their gifts of medicine power by controlling those that were weaker than them. Everyone was afraid of medicine people. In a community, people did not work together and there were many problems. Yamoria and his brother discussed the problems the people were encountering.

When they became adults, they travelled all over the north country, even into northern Alberta. Since they had observed how the people lived, they knew what to do. They split up and they each chose their own path to travel. Yamoria travelled in the Mackenzie Valley area. Yamagah chose the mountain range.

Yamoria could do many things very fast. He flew around the valley with his spirit medicine power and appeared wherever he wanted to be.

When Yamoria came across a large village, he would help the people complete their tasks fast. He had medicine power to control people's minds and he used this power for people to react fast. For example, if Yamoria wanted to hold a big meeting for all the village people, he just controlled their minds so that everyone would gather and everyone would run to the meeting place. Then he would stand in the middle of the crowd and talk.

He used his voice medicine power to speak to the people. When he spoke to the people with his voice medicine power, he spoke with a lot of authority and his speech was powerful. People were afraid of him when he spoke in this tone. He told the people about the kind of lifestyle they were leading and said it was not proper living; "You are people, human beings, and you should behave and conduct yourself like people all the time. I am going to establish a gathering place and I want everybody to go there to talk about any problems or concerns that you have.

"All the parents shall bring their children so they can listen as well. The Elders will go there to speak to the people. They will take turns speaking to the people. The Elders will be the main speakers at the gathering place. When you travel, use someone's tent as a gathering place even though as few as two families are travelling together. The Elders will talk about their past, from the beginning, about how the medicine people used to treat one another whether they were good or bad medicine-power people.

"By talking amongst yourselves, you will prevent and avoid a lot of problems from occurring again in the future. Only good things will come from such a gathering wherever you go. In order to accomplish this task, you have to work together as human beings and behave as mature adults. This gathering will teach you to govern yourselves.

"In a group, choose a person with medicine power to be your leader and listen to him. If that person does not turn out to be a good leader, choose another one. With a good leader you will learn to govern yourselves. You could talk about all these things in the gathering place."

These are the laws that he brought to the people:
1. Share with your people. If you kill a big game, share everything. Help the poor; help the Elders that are too old to work.
2. Help each other as much as possible. Help the sick people who are in need. Help them to get firewood. Cook for them and give them food.
3. When you lose someone in death, share your sorrow with the relatives of the one you lost. Help out widows and arrange for orphaned children.
4. Love each other as much as possible. Treat each other as brothers and sisters. Don't harm anyone.
5. Be respectful of Elders and everything around you. Don't run around when Elders are eating; sit down until they are finished.
6. Sleep at night and work during the day. Don't run around or laugh loudly when it gets dark. Everyone should sleep when darkness falls.
7. Be polite and don't argue with anyone. Don't harm anyone with your voice or actions.
8. Don't hurt anyone with your medicine power. Don't show your anger.
9. Young girls and boys should behave respectfully. Don't make fun of each other, especially in the matter of sex. Don't make fun of older men and women. Be polite to each other.
10. Pass on this teaching: Elders are to tell stories about the past, everyday. In this way, young people learn to distinguish between good and unacceptable behaviour. They will become the storytellers someday who will then keep the circle of life going.
11. Be happy at all times. The Creator has given you a great gift: Mother Earth. Take care of her and she will always give you food and shelter.
12. Don't worry. Just go about your work and make the best of

everything. Don't judge people. Find something good in everyone.
13. Don't lie about medicine power. Be honest at all times and have respect for medicine power.

"Prepare the children for a good life by teaching them in this way. It is your responsibility to do this," Yamoria said. This was the purpose of the gathering place that Yamoria spoke about: "Listen and obey the laws; live according to the laws and teach your children about the laws. It will serve as a guide for the children to live by and they will become good citizens from their teachings. If other people listen to those laws and live according to those laws, they will have a good life and be safe from bad medicine power."

Yamoria travelled to many villages. Things did not always go smoothly because there were many medicine-power people around trying to prevent him from doing good work. Many of these medicine-power people were wicked. Yamoria was aware of this and he confronted them at every turn.

Once, two men came forward to Yamoria and said, "We don't know who you are and we don't like people who come here telling us what to do." Yamoria knew that these two individuals were bad medicine men who were wicked, for they used their medicine power to murder people.

Yamoria clapped his hand and the two fellows instantly dropped to the ground and died. He told the bad medicine people that they had been killing people with their medicine power long enough: "You don't deserve to live amongst good people. It is better that you also die."

The people were really surprised to see Yamoria stand up to the bad medicine-power people. These two fellows were the ones that the people were most afraid of. From then on, everyone listened to Yamoria. The people were scared of Yamoria now, but they also had great respect for him. He spoke to them about many things—how to live as decent people and what kind of lifestyle they should lead.

He said, "The Creator put medicine power on earth for people to use it wisely so that they will have a good life, to help one another, to heal the sick and make them well. It is a terrible thing to kill someone with medicine power. I warn you people now not to harm anyone in the future with your medicine power. If you do, I will know about it immediately and take that medicine power away from you. Even if I am not nearby, I will still know about it.

"I want to stop medicine people from using their power to kill others. Medicine power is only to do good things, not to inflict harm on others. Love one another as much as you can. Treat each other with kindness and care. If you live by the laws I have given you, you will become good citizens to each other."

Many bad medicine-power people were angry with Yamoria and his teachings. Some even wanted to kill him. He was one man facing thousands of bad medicine-power men in the north. However, he was a *Beh Beh Tah*, and, therefore, he was able to overpower what other medicine-power people tried to do to him.

Yamoria succeeded in bringing the people together, to work together and to govern themselves. In time, Yamoria assisted and provided support to many people. He told people if they had a problem to come and see him and he would help them. People came to him from all over the country.

6: Yamagah, Brother of Yamoria

Both Yamagah and Yamoria travelled throughout the north. Yamagah travelled in the mountain area where many people lived and the game was plentiful. He got into trouble with a strong medicine man whose name was Eyonee Cho.

Eyonee Cho was a proud man, a leader and warrior for a large tribe. He was also a strong and powerful medicine-power man. When Yamagah came to his village, he started to mix with the people and talk to them about how they should live and conduct themselves. Eyonee Cho was not pleased to have a stranger coming into his village and teaching his people.

Eyonee Cho quarreled with Yamagah and a great conflict resulted. They even tried to kill one another using their medicine power, but they could not. It is likely that their medicine power was equally matched, which prevented both of them from being able to overpower the other man.

Yamagah married four women. Yamoria and Yamagah's lifestyle were completely different because of the way things happened in their lives. Wherever Yamagah went, people had great respect for him for they recognized him as a powerful medicine-power person. They made him a leader of a large tribe. Since he had four wives, Yamagah had many relatives. In no time at all, Yamagah had a large group of people who supported him as their leader. People were attracted to leaders who had strong medicine power. He protected the people and they ate well from his hunting.

Still, the conflict between Yamagah and Eyonee Cho was not resolved. They despised each other and were always thinking about how to have revenge on one another. One of the men would plan a raid on the other man's people, sneak into their camp when the warriors were not around, and kill their enemy. This was a common occurrence and it made it difficult for either group to grow larger.

One fall, when Yamagah was living in the mountain area, the men went hunting and left the women, children, and Elders behind in camp. They were gone for two weeks and were very successful. The snow was falling as they headed home with a large load of meat.

As they came upon a clearing, they startled a bear that attacked them in a rage. The men worked together to kill the angered animal, but, in the struggle, Yamagah was bitten in the arm. Before they could continue their journey, they bandaged Yamagah's wound and put his arm in a sling.

It was hot during the day and the men were sweaty from exertion. The weather grew colder as evening neared and their clothing froze. It was miserable conditions for all. Yamagah suggested that they make camp so they could dry their clothes and rest. Then they could head out early in the morning and be home before midday.

But the group had many young men who were anxious to get home. They wanted to keep going that night, so Yamagah went along with what the other men wanted.

Yamagah had a special nephew who he had left in camp. Whenever Yamagah returned to camp, he liked to play a game with him. As he approached the camp, he would yell out to his nephew and the boy would yell back. This time when Yamagah yelled out to his nephew, the boy did not respond. Something was wrong!

Yamagah whispered to the men, "I think the enemy is in our camp. Get ready to fight."

Suddenly, Eyonee Cho and his warriors burst from the bushes, screaming and running toward the men. They fought and fought. Yamagah and his men were tired from their long journey. They were no match for Eyonee Cho's group.

Yamagah fought bravely but was little help with his arm in a sling. He fled to the cliffs while the rest of his men were slaughtered. From the cliffs he could see the enemy burning everything they could not take with them. Before they left he yelled from his place of safety, "Before six years have passed you will see me and pay for what you have done to my family!"

Before long, Yamagah found another group of people who welcomed him. They immediately recognized him as a strong medicine man and were happy to make him their leader. All winter, Yamagah travelled all over inviting people to join his group. By spring of the next year he had a large group of followers.

All winter he planned his revenge against Eyonee Cho. In fact, he thought of little else. When summer arrived and the big game was fat, a large group of Eyonee Cho's men went hunting. Eyonee Cho also wanted to search for Yamagah's group and inflict his revenge.

After three days of searching, Yamagah found signs of hunters in the bush. His men soon discovered Eyonee Cho's camp. Eyonee Cho had a very large group of people in his camp with many tents. They were located in the valley of a high mountain where there were no trees. People in the camp would be able to see anyone approaching from a long ways away.

Yamagah was convinced that his men could sneak up near the camp unseen if they went during the drum dance that evening. There they waited until everyone had gone to their tent and fallen sleep. Yamagah used his medicine power to make sure they slept very deeply.

Then he overheard an old woman warning a young man, "Don't sleep too long. Yamagah promised to come back and have his revenge on us. Don't sleep too long!"

Soon Yamagah gave the signal and the men ran to the tent nearest them. Yamagah tore open the tent flap and screamed, "When you are young you're not supposed to sleep too long!" Then he clubbed the enemy in their beds. They never had a chance. Women grabbed their children and ran to the slope of the mountain.

When Yamagah witnessed the precious ones escaping to the mountainside, he yelled out his medicine-power command: "May all the people on the slope of the mountain turn back to rock!" And they did!

Soon there were no enemies left alive. Yamagah told his men, "Burn everything. I will track Eyonee Cho's brother and kill him myself. Wait for me here. I will return later today."

He flew with his spirit and quickly overtook the boy. He killed him right there. Then, with hatred in his heart, he dragged the boy's slain body and threw him over a tree stump where the birds would eat him. He smiled when he thought of the horror Eyonee Cho would feel when

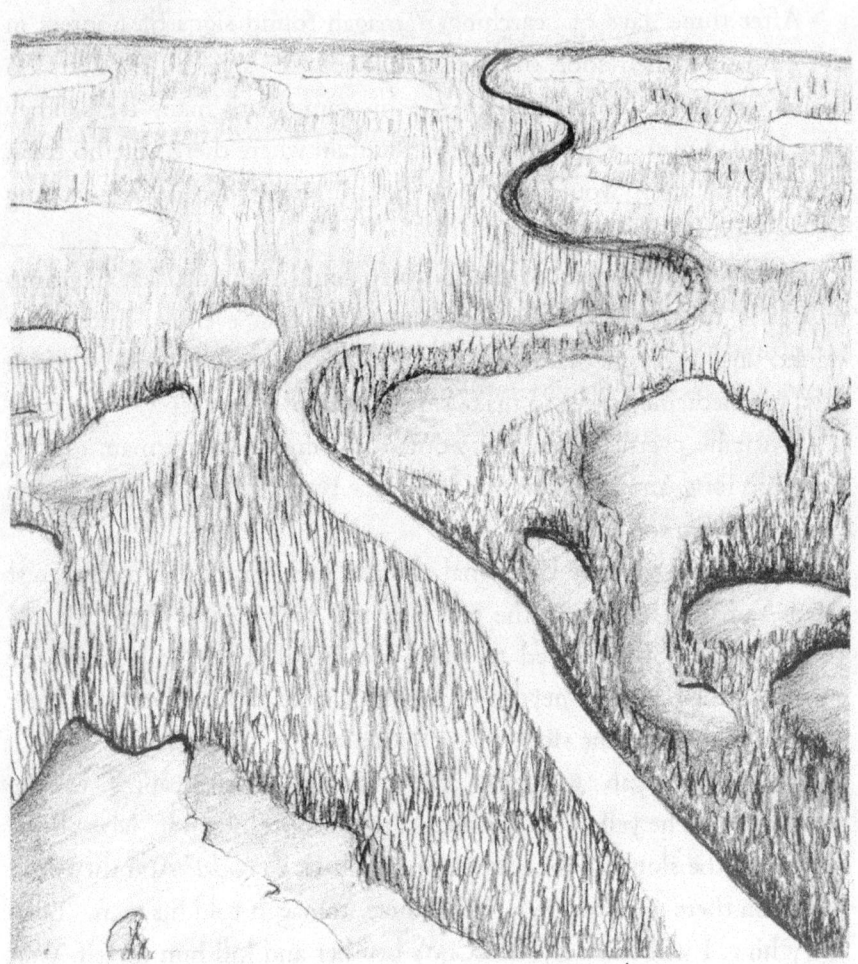

he saw his younger brother this way.

Then Yamagah walked away from the hunting trail to the side of a small creek. He made a small fire there and cooked something to eat. Then he laid down to rest and fell right asleep.

Meanwhile, Eyonee Cho was returning from a hunting trip with a heavy pack of meat. He was walking along the hunting trail when he noticed the camp dogs howling. This puzzled him. He wondered, "Yamagah promised to come back and pay me a visit. Is that why the dogs are howling?"

He travelled down the trail at a quicker pace, anxious to see his family safe and sound. When he turned a bend he saw many birds on a tree stump. He put his pack down and went over to investigate. There was his younger brother whom he loved, dead and ravaged by the scavengers!

Instantly, he knew: "Yamagah! When I see him, I will kill him with my bare hands!"

Gently, he placed his brother's body on the ground. He thought, "I wonder if anyone else is alive. Why bother carrying this heavy pack of meat? Maybe there is no one left to feed."

Then he took the meat and placed it on top of his brother's body and covered it with rocks. He continued down the trail until he noticed the smell of smoke. He searched the area with his eyes and noticed a small fire. Silently he crept near. There was his enemy: Yamagah, sleeping in the hot sun. Eyonee Cho took a club to smash his head into the rocks. Just as he raised the club, Yamagah opened his eyes and grabbed him.

The two men fought and fought, but because their medicine power was equal, neither could win. After many hours they sat apart from each other, exhausted but ready if the other should strike again.

Then Eyonee Cho spoke, "It seems neither of us can destroy the other no matter how badly we want to. We cannot fight like this forever. Now what will we do?"

Yamagah said, "If you want to talk peace now, I am prepared to listen."

Eyonee Cho answered, "We are not too old yet. Maybe we could still do some good for the people. It will take a long time for our anger to go away, but if we try, maybe we can forgive each other someday. Maybe even learn to love each other."

Yamagah smiled, "As long as I live, I will never learn to hug or kiss a man as ugly as you, so don't even think about it. You're right though. When I was young, my brother, Yamoria, and I planned to travel the country. We wanted to help people to live better lives, to work together, and govern ourselves. That was our plan. But we took different paths. As soon as I met you we began to fight, and it has continued to this day. You and I have lived a violent life full of hatred and revenge. It is our fault, both you and me. Maybe you're right. Maybe it's not too late to do something good for the people. I agree that we should live in peace."

They sat silently with each other for a long time. Then Yamagah asked, "Why don't you come home with me. There is nothing for you here now. Maybe you will find a wife someday among my people and have a good life again. You know, we could live in one tent. Then we will have to let go of our anger toward each other."

They shook hands and walked back to Eyonee Cho's camp. Yamagah's men were still there waiting for him. They were surprised to see the two men calmly walking beside each other. They looked at Yamagah puzzled.

He chose his words carefully: "This man will be coming with us. He is to be treated with kindness and respect. If you think you want to attack him, forget it! I have been fighting him all day and I have not been able to harm him. He is too powerful. I have invited him to live among us. If you do anything against him, then you also do it against me."

After three days of travelling, they returned to Yamagah's camp. Many people felt anger and bitterness toward Eyonee Cho because of his past acts of violence and the deaths he caused of people they loved. However, Yamagah made it very clear that he was to be treated fairly. The people respected Yamagah, so they followed his wishes even though they did not like it. People were afraid of the two men but also knew that their strong medicine power could help them to survive both famine and war. This was important to everyone.

Today there are many shapes in the rock of the mountain slope that we believe are the mothers and children who fled to the mountainside. Some rocks look like a woman with a baby on her back. Others look like a woman holding the hand of a child. Of course, this is what they are.

7: Yamagah: the Story Continues...

Yamagah and Eyonee Cho had medicine power for everything, even wildlife. They were very successful with hunting and fishing. They controlled a large herd of caribou that migrated from the arctic coast to the mountains each year. They made sure that part of the herd always travelled near their camp. They also taught the people how to treat the caribou with respect.

In this era, young women looking for a husband found men with medicine power very attractive. They were sure that a man with gifts for hunting, fishing, and trapping would be able to provide for them and their children. Then they would have a good life.

For this reason, Eyonee Cho was considered a "good catch" in the community, and all the single women were chasing him. When he did marry, instead of moving into a tent with his new wife, he remained in the tent with Yamagah and his wives. Yamagah had taken four wives by this time and he had many children. It was quite a family!

Soon they had a large tent made. It was the biggest tent in the country, consisting of thirty moose-hides. Eventually, Eyonee Cho also had four wives and his own children. The eight women that were married to the two men were all strong women in their own right. They cooked and sewed for the big family very well. Together, the women eventually developed a system for how people should work together. They were powerful examples to the community of how to get along with others and help each other.

At that time, there were no Dene laws, so the two leaders set up a system in which the Elders taught the children each day in a gathering place. Here they learned how to be good citizens of the community and how to live in harmony together. They also learned many skills that they would need all their lives.

It was very busy in the tent, especially when all the group's children and Elders gathered there each day for teaching. This was a form of Dene school, actually. It was miraculous how the whole group functioned without conflicts and problems.

Yamagah and Eyonee Cho also taught by example that a person can overcome their own hatred toward someone and choose to love them and work in co-operation with them instead.

The two men used their medicine power to monitor whether any other medicine people were using their powers to harm others. When they found out that a medicine person had—especially if that person had killed another—they took action. They ended the lives of a few medicine people for doing this, and they warned the rest, "If anyone of you kills someone using medicine power, we will know and make sure that your life is ended as well."

Many people from far away places came to join their group. It was a good life for them with abundant food and other resources, as well as co-operation and harmony among the people. They soon became the largest nation in the area.

The two men lived so long that they outlived all their wives who had died of old age. They had over forty grandchildren, and still they lived together. By this time they no longer needed a big tent so they lived in a small one with four grandchildren to look after them. Some say they lived to one hundred and fifty years old. They were blind, could not hear much of anything, and had lost all their hair. Their skin was very white by then, and they were skinny. They could no longer walk and crawled to move about their tent. They spent most of their time mumbling to anyone who would visit, but no one paid them much attention anymore.

Then one day, while one of the grandchildren was busy outside, they talked between themselves. Eyonee Cho said, "When I was walking home one day with a great, heavy pack of meat I was very pleased with myself. Then I heard the dogs howling in the distance. I thought of Yamagah and remembered that he had promised to come and attack us someday. I wondered if he had come."

Then, from across the tent, Yamagah yelled, "Old man, what are you talking about!"

Eyonee Cho answered, "I'm talking about the time you killed my brother!" Next thing you know, the two feeble, old men were fighting each other. They had no medicine power by this time, so they tried to hit each other but their skinny arms just fell. They tried to scratch, but they had no fingernails; they tried to bite, but they had no teeth. The granddaughter came in and easily stopped the fight.

The old foes lay on their blanket for a long while. Later that day, they told their grandchildren to tell everyone to come and visit them. "We have something to tell them," they said.

Soon everyone was there. And an Elder said, "We all came as you have requested. What is it that you two men want to tell us?"

The old men took turns talking. They described what they had tried to do in their lives. Then they said, "We have lived long enough. We will die now. Bury us on that high hill. In the future, Dene will bring their children to that place to sleep, and if the Creator chooses, they will receive medicine power."

Soon after, both men died as they had said.

8: Medicine-Power Law

As with all things, medicine power has its own laws that govern its use. When the world was new, Aboriginal people were gifted with many, many medicine people and our mere survival depended on the proper use of medicine power. Therefore, our people were careful to follow these laws and avoid problems, even though it required great self-discipline. Animals also have medicine power and are required to follow the same laws.

For a medicine person, following the rules and obeying the law at all times is of the utmost importance. For Christians, the church provides the law of the Church. It is really the law of the Creator. One law of the church is to confess your sins to a priest and your sins will be forgiven. The purpose of the law is to receive forgiveness. If a medicine-power person confessed the wrong things he did using medicine power, I believe the kind Creator would forgive that individual.

I believe that a crime committed using medicine power is one of the worst possible crimes. Still, it is not my place to say that a medicine-power crime cannot be forgiven. There has to be a way for all crimes to be forgiven somehow. I ask myself, "What did we do before the Europeans came and brought the priests to us?" I can't believe that our people died without being forgiven for our sins just because we didn't have a priest with whom to say confession.

As I have discussed, Yamoria established Dene laws. He taught a way of life that brought harmony and happiness to the people. One of the teachings that the people followed everyday involved storytelling. Each night, after the work of the day was completed and just before bed, the people would gather together and the Elders would tell stories. They would also teach how to live a good life and be a responsible and valued member of the community. This even happened when they were travelling all over the bush and with as little as two families.

When the world was new there was very little sickness. It was common to live to one hundred years old and, therefore, there were many Elders willing to fill this role as teachers and the carriers of wisdom, history, and stories. This was a very effective system.

Yamoria also taught parents to bring their children to a gathering place every day to listen to Elders teach. At that time, medicine power was extremely valuable and every parent wanted his or her child to have medicine power. It was common for parents to go to great lengths to try to obtain medicine power for their child. They knew that medicine power would only come to a person with a strong mind and good heart. As soon as their child began to talk, they would take her or him to learn from the Elders about how to become a good person. Establishing a place for the people to gather each day was an essential aspect of Dene life.

Parents, curious to know whether or not their child possessed medicine power, could also approach a medicine person and ask him or her to perform a ceremony. Some parents, upon discovering that their child did have medicine power, would ask another medicine person to find out what kind of medicine power it was. However, this is difficult to determine for most medicine people, and, often, parents just had to wait until their child matured. To hear your child was born with medicine power was a joyous event!

Here is a story about parents who sacrificed and worked very hard for their children to obtain medicine power.

There was a good family who lived according to medicine-power laws. Although they had worked very hard for their children to obtain medicine power, their son, at thirty years old, and daughter, at twenty years old, still had not received any medicine power. The family had even spent many years living in isolation, away from large groups of people, to protect their children from bad influences that could ruin their chances of obtaining medicine power.

From the time they were born, their parents, in hopes their children would receive medicine power, taught them carefully. They used tools for medicine power, such as the drum, and songs to help their children. They took them to sacred places where other young people had received medicine power. None of these things worked.

Finally, the father had a talk with the son: "There must be something preventing you from receiving medicine power. Perhaps you have done something wrong or had bad thoughts? The Creator created everything on Mother Earth, the stars in the sky and all things. The Creator also made medicine power for us to help us live. A few very fortunate people receive medicine power from the Creator before they are born. They don't have to work for it. They are very lucky. Then there are individuals like you who have tried and tried for thirty years and you still do not have any medicine power.

"We have tried everything. The only thing I can think of now is that something is preventing you from receiving medicine power.

"Tonight, somewhere, our people are gathering, as they do all the time. Elders are teaching how to live a good life and how to pray to the Creator. You know, I have often thought that we should organize ourselves to pray to the Creator. If we all came together to pray and beg the Creator for what we need, our prayers would be so much stronger. Instead we pray, each of us, alone. Perhaps that is why it seems the Creator does not listen.

"Long ago, Yamoria lived among our people. His life is legendary. I believe he was sent by the Creator to help us because we were living such a pitiful existence up until that time. He taught us how to work and live together as human beings should. He's the one who taught us to gather each day to listen to the Elders teach us how to live a good life. It is so important to have great respect for all that the Creator has made for us."

For Dene people, we understand that all things have a spirit. Our many medicine people have told us this. When a medicine person prays, they will often talk to the spirit of various things in creation and ask for help from them. For example, if a medicine person has medicine power for the mountains, he or she could communicate with the spirit of the mountains. That spirit may even take a human-like form to allow for easier communication. Anyone can talk to the spirits of things, but they may not be able to understand what the spirit says back. When a medicine person who has medicine power for the mountains talks to it, he or she understands what the spirit of the mountain is saying back.

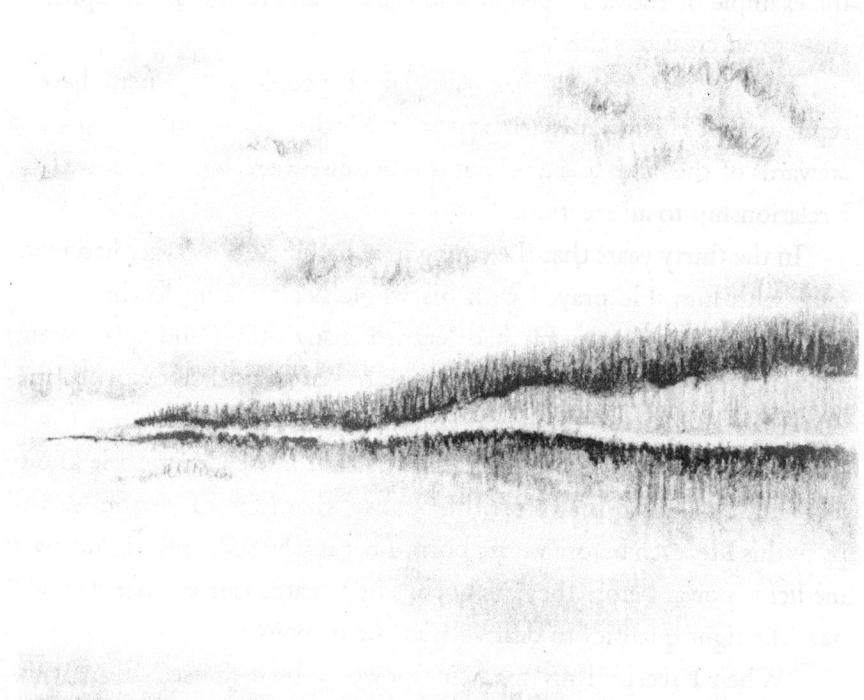

I have witnessed my parents greet the mountains, lakes, the sun, and the moon in this way. They would stand and shout out to them asking for their help. I remember feeling foolish at the time because I was just a boy and could not understand how they could communicate with the mountain. Still, all Dene people who travel on the land follow the example of medicine people and honour and recognize the spirit of these great creations this way.

This is one reason that Aboriginal people everywhere have a reputation for living in harmony with Mother Earth and being good stewards of the land. It is true, but it is because we recognize that we have a relationship to all creation.

In the thirty years that the young man had lived, his father had many talks with him. He prayed with his whole heart asking for his son to receive medicine power. He had learned many things and spent many, many nights at gathering places listening to Elders teach about medicine-power law and how to be a good citizen.

He told his son, "Nothing is impossible for the Creator. He knows all things, including the future. He knows what kind of person we will be in this life, even before we are born. That is why some people are given medicine power before they are born. The Creator can see that they will have the right qualities to deal with medicine power.

"When I received my medicine power, a man dressed all in white appeared to me. I believe he was a helper sent from the Creator. You know, it is possible that even if you have done something wrong in this life that the Creator would forgive you and still give you medicine power. I would like to try one more thing. If this does not work, then we will give up and you will live your life without medicine power. It will be a sad thing because it means you will be poor and have to depend on others all your life. But we will accept it.

"I want you to go to that spot we camped last year by the big lake. Stay there for five days and pray to the Creator the best way you know how. You can even use plain language and tell the Creator what is in your heart and mind and what you are asking for from him. Then return here on the fifth day.

"In the meantime, I will use my medicine power for the canoe and make a brand new canoe for you. You will be the first person to set foot inside it."

The old man built the canoe and his son went to the lake. After five days, the canoe was built and ready, but the boy came back without any power of any kind. So the old man told the boy to take the canoe and paddle along the shore and go back to the camp. He was to sleep out there for one more night.

The young man took the canoe, a bow and arrow, and his spear, and then paddled along the lakeshore. Soon he saw a group of islands and a woodland caribou. He chased the caribou and caught up to it while it was still swimming. Then he struck it with his spear, tied a rope to it, and pulled it onto shore. Right there he began to cut up the meat. He built a nice fire to cook the caribou head, which he hung next to the fire.

Soon afterward, a powerful feeling came over him and, try as he might, he could not stay awake. As soon as his head touched the ground, he fell asleep and a vision appeared to him. An old man was sitting on a large leaf floating on the water. He came ashore and approached the young man. He said, "My grandson, what are you doing here? I want to go across the lake where two bad boys took my wife. Will you come with me and help me? It won't take long."

The young man looked at the old man and then at the caribou head that he was cooking. He replied, "I would like to help you, but, as you can see, I am cooking this caribou."

The old man assured him that it wouldn't take long and the young man agreed. "Before we go," said the old man, "why don't you tell me about this thing that you have done wrong?"

"But, Grandfather," the young man said, "I have not done a single thing wrong in my whole life. I have worked very hard to listen to my parents and Elders."

The old man looked at him with piercing eyes. Finally, when the young man could not stand his gaze any longer the old man said, "I will help you, if you cannot remember.

"Long ago, one spring, there was still a little snow on the ground. You got up to make a fire. It was quiet with no wind and you could hear very well. As you were making the fire your sister got up and went outside to relieve herself. It was so quiet that you heard your sister relieve herself and you had thoughts about her that are not right to think about your sister. Is what I'm saying true?"

The boy looked down at the ground and said in a quiet voice, "Yes, it is true. Now you have reminded me. I did do something wrong."

The old man's eyes became kindly again. "It is good that you have finally admitted this thing you have done wrong. Still, you are forgiven. I know you have worked very hard. In fact, I do believe no one has worked harder. Now that you have admitted this to me, you can come with me," the old man said.

Then he jumped on the big leaf and motioned for the young man to get on behind him. In what seemed like two strokes of the paddle, they were across the lake. They went ashore where a village was visible. Just then people from the village started yelling the young man's name and shouting for him to visit them. The old man told him, "I will wait here for you. Go and see them. They will give you all the medicine power you will need in this life."

That is exactly what they did. The young man received medicine power for fishnets and fishhooks, to hunt big game, and all the powers he needed to survive well on Mother Earth. Then he returned to where the old man was waiting.

"I will go get your grandmother now," said the old man. They walked over to the end of the village. One boy came up to the old man threatening to fight with him, but in an instant the grandfather picked up the boy and threw him to the ground. The pitiful boy's body was sticking half in the ground and half out. Then he went for the other boy and threw him up in the air. He got stuck in a big tree and that was where he stayed.

The man collected his wife and headed back to the young man's camp where the caribou head was still cooking. The old man gave him some last instructions: "When you go, just take the caribou jaw back with you and try to get home early before anyone sees you. When you reach camp, go straight to your bed. You will see that I am right beside you. Then I will give you medicine power to sing and you will own all the medicine power that everyone has given you."

The young man woke up suddenly to see the caribou head still turning. He followed the grandfather's instruction and received many items of medicine power that day, in an instant. Then the young man became a strong singer and his family was very happy to have another medicine man in the family.

9: THE STORY OF EDWAR

EDWAR WAS A GREAT MEDICINE MAN WHO LIVED IN 1850. HE CAME from Aklavik, NWT, and was a member of the Gwich'in tribe. Edwar was a private man who didn't discuss his medicine power publicly. Still, in time, many, many people asked Edwar to help them with their problems.

As it happened, this was the time that the first Europeans ever came into the north. The fur traders arrived initially; then the missionaries came, intent on converting the people to Christianity. Each priest wore striking attire: a long black coat with a large cross on his belt. Our people were afraid of these strange men. They thought they must be the most powerful of medicine men.

But Edwar was not afraid of powerful medicine men. He was not afraid of anyone. He decided he wanted to visit and talk to this man they called "priest." Edwar explained to the priest that he possessed a great deal of medicine power, although he had never asked for this power. He also told the priest that he found the constant requests for help overwhelming and difficult. He sought a way to rid himself of his medicine power.

He said, "I have heard people talk about you. They say you are a most powerful medicine person and that you can send people to heaven or hell after they die. I have also heard that you tell people that medicine power comes from an evil spirit you call 'Devil' and you don't like it. This is why I have come to you for help, to get rid of my medicine power. It's not my fault that I have too much. It was given to me before I was born.

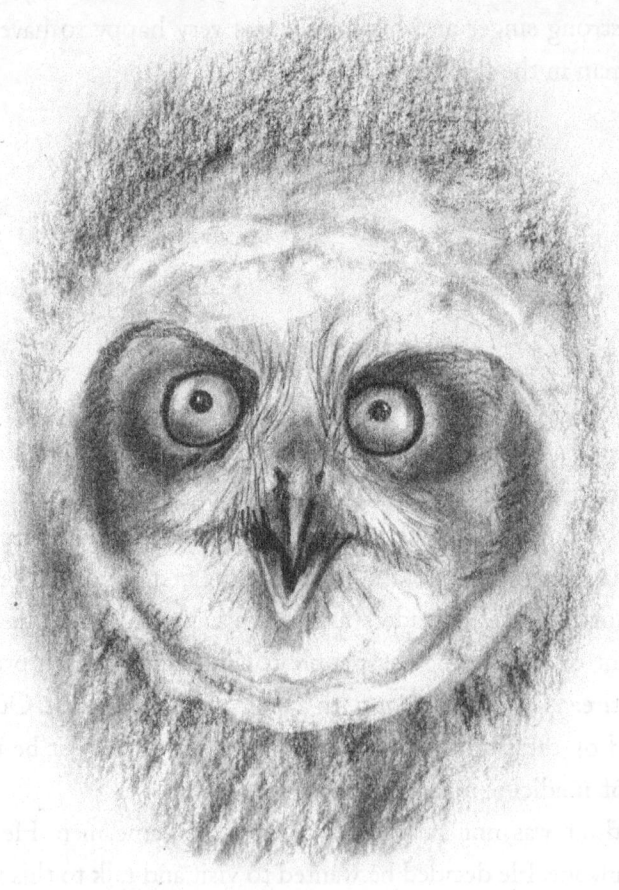

But I don't care for the life of a medicine man. It's a difficult life dealing with everyone's problems."

The priest truly had no knowledge of medicine power. Even the Dene people who had lived with medicine power for the last one hundred thousand years understood very little about medicine power. Still, the priest thought he could tell Edwar how to rid himself of his many gifts. The priest smiled and said, "Edwar, this is an easy thing that you ask of me. Simply kneel here in front of me and confess to me all the medicine power you possess. Then I will pray over you and all your medicine power will be gone in an instant."

Edwar looked at the priest in surprise and said, "I didn't think it was that easy." He told the priest, "If what you say is true, do I have to confess everything to get rid of my medicine power?"

The priest said, "Yes, you have to confess everything."

Edwar sat quietly for a moment. Then he looked at the priest and said, "I have a lot of medicine power. I don't use it unless I must. Most of the medicine power spirits are just there waiting to work through me but I ignore them. If I have to confess each item one by one it will take a very long time. You see, I have medicine power for space, the sun, moon, stars, and all the planets in space. I also have medicine for the northern lights, wind, fog, clouds, air, and all things that cover the earth. Then the earth also, all life in the water, in the air, all the insects that crawl on the earth, the plants, trees, rocks, mountains, rivers, landslides, earthquakes, rain, lightning, thunder, snow, and anything to do with weather.

"As you can see, there are many, many items. If I have to confess them one by one, I could do that if that is what's necessary. But I think I will be kneeling down in front of you day after day for about two to three years. Of course, then I will have to live in your house and eat from your table until we are finished."

The priest responded with shock and anger, "You cannot do that. I am poor and I can't look after you!"

"But" said Edwar, "I thought you said it was easy to do."

The priest suddenly regained his composure and explained, "You are a powerful man, Edwar. I don't know what to say to you. All I can do is pray over you and give you the best advice that I can." Then he suggested, "Why don't you kneel here in front of me and I will pray over you."

When he was done he said to Edwar, "Go home and pray to God as much as you can. Try to be a normal person and forget that you ever owned medicine power." Edwar went home, still possessing the power as before. Nothing had changed for Edwar.

When the world was new, there were many medicine people who had received medicine power just like in Edwar's case. The Creator gave them their medicine power all at once, instead of using a messenger for each item of medicine power.

Another story of Edwar that would best illustrate this is the time he was with about three families with children and Elders. One of the men in the camp had shot a moose about ten miles in the bush, so the families packed and travelled to where the moose was shot to eat when they arrived. But there was a huge problem: a forest fire had crept up on the area and high winds blew the flames around them.

The people grew worried. Suddenly, the trees around them started to smoke and burst into flames. Some said they were going to be burned alive. One of the Elders yelled to Edwar over the roar of the flames, "You call yourself a medicine man. Do something!"

Edwar had to raise his voice to be heard. He yelled, "The spirit of the wind—change now! Blow away from us right now!" The wind did change. Edwar yelled again, "Spirit of thunder—pour down a lot of rain right now." A black cloud appeared in the sky. You could hear thunder and it rained a lot. Edwar yelled at the people, "Go to sleep now!" The people immediately fell asleep. In the morning, there was sunshine. There was no fire, no wind. So, Edwar did that for his people. He was a great man.

10: THE STORY OF KENNY

KENNY CAME FROM DÉLINE, NWT, AND LIVED DURING THE SAME period as Edwar. His good friend—my grandfather, Paul Blondin—once asked him to explain how he used medicine power to play hand games. This was the first time Kenny ever talked about his medicine power in public and we can learn a great deal from his teachings.

In 1870, people travelled far and wide to trade furs at Déline. This was the only trading post for the whole area of the Great Bear Lake, the mountain region up to the Yukon border, and all the Mackenzie River area.

Kenny was quite different from most medicine people. He was a very quiet man who spent most of his time alone. He was not known for talking about his medicine power at all and, as a result, few people knew him or sought out his help. Also, Kenny had never played hand games in his whole life until the day he and Paul Blondin and the others came into Fort Ross with a sled full of furs.

The Elders had convinced Paul to travel to a trading post called Fort Ross to trade their furs, even though this outpost was seven hundred miles away across the mountains. They had heard from the Mountain Dene that their country was infested with people from all over the world who were searching for gold. This also brought lots of business to the area and a number of stores had opened. The traders were known for paying top prices for furs, far more than in Déline. They also had rifles for sale that shot shells, which was a great improvement over the muzzleloader guns they were using.

Paul found seven men and their families, including his son, to go with him on this journey. He had heard that the people of the Yukon Territory used medicine power to play hand games. This worried Paul somewhat, even though he had medicine power that could help him win at hand games himself. Paul had medicine power that could see an object in a closed hand. He told himself that he could use this medicine power to play hand games if he had to.

Then Paul remembered that his friend, Kenny, also had medicine power that would be useful in hand games. He decided that Kenny must accompany him to the Yukon. He approached Kenny and asked him to join him on the journey, but Kenny was reluctant. Kenny said, "I would like to go with you, Paul, but it is a long trip and I've got no money."

Then Paul reassured him, "Listen, Kenny, if you join me I'll give you five marten that you can use to buy things when we get there." This convinced Kenny and off they went. In about forty-five days they finally arrived in Fort Ross, Yukon Territory.

It was common for the people of Déline to meet the Mountain people of Fort Ross, and so they weren't complete strangers to each other. The Mountain people welcomed their guests and the two groups visited amiably with each other. One of the Elders from Fort Ross warned the visitors, "It is unfortunate, but there is a large group of people who are travelling around this country who are up to no good. They visit each of the small villages in our territory where they gamble at hand games and poker. They win but only because they cheat by using medicine power. Of course, it is not fair, and it's foolish to use medicine power to play a friendly match of hand games. I would advise you to avoid playing with these people if they come here."

Two days after the Elder's warning, a large group of people arrived at the fort. They were sixty people in all, with thirty dog teams and two people on each toboggan. What a noise they made! After they had eaten, the leader of their group said, "We don't see each other everyday. Let's have some fun! The white people have a good custom. When they greet each other they take a bottle of whiskey and have a friendly drink. But, us Indians, we don't have whiskey. It is not our custom to drink. We have other ways to make ourselves happy. Tea dances and hand games—that is our culture. We heard there are some people from Déline visiting here. I would like to talk to the leader of that group."

Paul Blondin stood up. With a medicine-power spirit voice he bellowed, "What do you want to talk about?" The sound and strength of his voice was startling, and the other man shuddered. Then Paul said, "Oh, let's have some fun and be happy. I want to challenge you and your people to a hand-games match."

Paul thought it would be wise to follow the Elder's advice so he replied, "Oh, we are from the Mackenzie Valley and we don't know how to play hand games. Sorry, but we cannot play this game with you."

But the other man would not be dismissed so easily. He said, "I am surprised that a man like you doesn't know how to play hand games. I think you must be lying about that. You're probably just scared of me. Hear that, everybody? This man from the Mackenzie Valley is scared to play hand games with me."

The man's taunt was successful in angering Paul. He replied, "Since my mother put me on this Earth, I have been afraid of no one, and I sure am not afraid of you. You want to play hand games? Fine, let's play." So the man shouted to his people, "Get the drums! We're going to play hand games!"

The people from Fort Ross had never played with the people from Déline before. There were sixty men on the Yukon team but only eight men on the Déline team. They had ten drums and the game started right up.

In hand games, one player from each team attempts to guess in which hand each of his opponents has hidden an object. When the player guesses right, that person hiding the object is kicked out of that match. When all of the players on one team have been kicked out of the match, they switch roles and one player from the other team attempts to guess in which hand each of his opponents has hidden an object.

Right from the start, the team from Fort Norman began to lose. Paul and his son, Edward Blondin, had a good cache of money from the furs they had sold, but the rest of the men and their families were poor. They had no money, so they wagered with matches, shells, and plug tobacco. They paid with whatever they had. After an hour and a half, they had lost four games. It seemed that they would lose everything they had. That was when Paul started to worry about his group. He knew he had medicine power that could help him win at hand games, but he had only used it twice before in his whole life. He preferred to play friendly hand games without medicine power; still, he knew the other team was winning because they were using medicine power. He felt compelled to protect his people.

He took Kenny aside to talk about this problem. "You know, Kenny," he said quietly, "that other team is using medicine power to win. I'm worried that we're not going to have anything left in a couple more hours if we don't do something. We won't even have our dog teams to go home with and then we'll be stuck here. Kenny, you are my friend. You are like a brother to me. We are the same age. We grew up together and played together every day of our lives. I want to ask your help with something. I know you have medicine power for hand games and that's why you never play hand games with your own people. I'm right, aren't I? Please help your people here today. Play hand games with us. Help us to win."

Kenny shook his head, "Well, my friend. I cannot play hand games myself, but I'll tell you what I'll do. I will send my twelve-year-old to play for me. I'll sit behind him and tell him what to do. Go inside. I will come right away. I want to find an object for the boy to play with. Then I'll be right there."

Kenny found a small cone from a spruce tree. When he and the boy entered the tent the game was already in play. As expected, the Yukon team was still winning. Paul could see that there were three people on the Yukon team with medicine power who always played to the last.

Paul had special medicine power to control people's minds, but he didn't use this power on his people as he considered it cruel to make people do what you want through medicine power. He had heard the many stories of powerful medicine men that had the same gift of medicine power. Some of them, like Yamoria, used their medicine power over people's minds for good, but others took advantage of this gift and used it for their own purposes. He did not want to ever become like them. Reluctantly, he decided he must use this gift to help his people.

Paul took one of his team members aside. This was the man who had been attempting to guess where the objects were hidden. He said, "When these three people are the last ones left to guess, just like what has happened in all the other matches, let me take a turn at guessing. I have a plan."

Then, just as Paul had suggested, there were only three players left on the other team. Paul exchanged places with the man who had been guessing. Paul knelt down in front of his opponents. Once again, they put their hands under the blanket. The other men were banging very loud and quick on the drums and the crowd was very excited to see what would happen with a new man guessing. Finally, the three men thrust their closed fists forward looking straight ahead, careful not to reveal which hand hid the object.

Paul pointed his finger to the left, which meant that he guessed that all three of them had the object in their left hand. Each man slowly opened his left hand to reveal the object. The crowd went wild with excitement! After all those matches, the Déline team had finally guessed right for the last three men.

Then it was the Déline team's turn to hide the objects. Kenny's little boy sat in a row on the ground with the rest of the men. Kenny sat right behind him. The Yukon team's player guessed and guessed each round but he could not catch the little boy. The Déline team won and won. Finally, Kenny whispered to his boy, "Don't open your hand. Just pretend that he guessed right and the game will be over." This is what the boy did, even though they still did not guess right.

Then Paul got up and faced the leader of the Yukon team. He told them, "You should have quit when I told you I didn't know how to play hand games. Now your people have lost plenty. I only said that because I didn't want to play against a team that uses medicine power to win.

But, still, I thought we would play for three or four days. Here we are a few hours later and you're ready to quit. Maybe you are scared of me, my friend."

Everyone stood still and listened when they heard Paul's challenge.

The Yukon leader said, "I'll admit it. I am scared of you. It's been a long time since anyone has beaten us at hand games. Let's quit while we are still friends and there are no hard feelings between us." The two men shook hands and the games were over.

In a short time, the group from Déline began the long journey back home. Along the way, they shot a moose and made camp so they could rest and have a good meal. After everyone had eaten their fill, they gathered in a big tent to joke and laugh and tell stories. They were happy without a worry.

REGARDING PAUL BLONDIN

Blondin is not the right name for Paul, but I can't find the first name he was born with. I believe Paul came from a different family. Paul is my dad's father. Paul married Edwar's daughter. Their first son is my dad. I believe Edwar Blondin was born in 1910. My dad was the first-born boy in the family. Following Dene culture, the first-born boy slept with his grandfather in hopes that he would inherit his grandfather's medicine. So, Edward Blondin, as a boy, slept with his grandfather, Edwar, for two years. That is how he inherited his name. That is why he was called Edward Blondin. Also, he inherited his medicine power from Edwar—not much, but some. *Blondin* is not really a name from the Dene people. When Edwar was a kid, he trapped with private trappers from Ottawa for two years. The trappers died, so Edwar inherited the name "Blondin" from them. The name stuck a long way into the future.

11: SPACE AND THE PLANETS

HERE IS A STORY OF KENNY'S TEACHING ABOUT THE SUN, THE MOON, and the planets. At that time, 1910, the Dene people of the area did not have scientific knowledge of outer space. It was much later in history, after contact with the Europeans, that we learned what scientists had discovered about the planets. Dene people tried to live their lives according to the teaching that said, "Be as happy as possible because life is short."

For the most part, we were not interested in learning about things that did not concern us. We were happy the way we were. The sun came up. The sun went down. The moon is there as light in the night. The land is here and takes care of us. This was enough to know and understand. Kenny's teaching did not make a big impression on the people that night. But it seems to have made a big impression on Paul Blondin, because he remembered and passed this story on to our people.

One night, Paul Blondin asked Kenny, "My friend, my brother, something has been bothering me that I've been meaning to ask you about. It seems that medicine power is getting weak in this country. They say when the world was new there were many, many powerful medicine people. It's not like that anymore. We are getting to be so few. We own a small amount of medicine power, whatever it may be, but are taught that we cannot talk about our own medicine power. I was told not to talk about my own medicine power because it could hurt other people who have medicine power. I suppose that is why most medicine people don't speak about it. But, you know, I have this crazy idea that this is wrong. I think that you can talk about medicine power and it won't hurt anyone. Anyhow, my friend, please tell me how you used your medicine power to beat that Yukon team."

Kenny was moved by Paul Blondin's questions. He said, "I have never talked about my medicine power to anyone in my whole life. To tell you the truth, it's kind of scary for me. That is why I've been such a quiet person all my life, I think. My medicine power is very different than other people's. I will tell you a story.

"Before I was born, an old man dressed in white appeared to me. He said to me, 'I have come to give you medicine power for the sun and the nine planets, including Mother Earth. They will be your partners. Together you will be able to do good things.'

"For a long time, I could not understand how to use my own medicine power. I was poor. I didn't have medicine power for moose or caribou or fish to help me eat well. I was pitiful at times. Finally, I explored space to learn how all these planets worked. Once I saw the moon and the stars playing hand games. After that, I didn't want to play hand games with my own people and I never did.

"The sun is my partner and I understand how it operates. It is very big, the sun. You think Mother Earth is big? The sun is five times bigger. You could fit five of our Earths into the Sun. It's very far away. That is why it's so small. It's just a burning ball of fire.

"Here on earth we burn wood, oil, and coal. But the sun burns something different that we never saw here on earth. The sun itself is not just a fire. The substance is rock. Over time, small particles break away, which are then used as fuel for the fire. It also burns something similar to air that the sun sucks in and burns. The vast space is full of it, so the sun will never run out of fuel. It could burn forever. Also, the sun doesn't move at all. It just stays in one place and burns fuel. The sun is a very important planet in space.

"It helps Mother Earth and creates both winter and summer here on earth. The heat we enjoy is from the sun. My partner, the sun, and I still talk to each other. Once, the sun said we could change the weather and make it warmer in the cold winter. But I have never tried it."

Kenny kept on talking all night. Some people were unimpressed and fell asleep, but Paul Blondin and my dad, Edward Blondin, were very interested. It was the first time they had ever heard anyone explain about the planets and space.

My dad told these stories to me. He said, "We used to think everything was moving in the sky, but now I know it is not so. It is Mother Earth that is moving. Also, the moon is not as far away as the sun. It is between the earth and sun. It does not move and it's just a block of rock and sand." Kenny once told him, "I was there and walked on the moon. The moon is my partner, too. I can talk to the moon as well. You understand that this does not mean I travelled there with my physical body. I mean I travelled there with my spirit. That is how I can travel in space."

Kenny explained, "Mother Earth is not alone in space. There are nine planets in this vast space and Mother Earth is one of them. Each planet is spinning. Mother Earth spins so fast that even water stays on it. If she did not spin, the water would spill out into space and we would die. Mother Earth is turning so fast that we don't even know it. It makes one whole revolution in a day. Some people think the sun goes up and down, but it's not like that. Mother Earth is revolving. When the place we are standing on is facing the sun, it is day. When Mother Earth turns and we are on the opposite side away from the sun, it is night. It takes one whole year for the Earth to travel in a great circle around the sun."

Kenny reflected, "It is amazing how all these planets follow the same route around the sun for thousands of years. It doesn't vary from that route. It is just like a trail for the planets. If Mother Earth varied from her route, we would all die.

"You know that the stars are just big rocks floating out in space. Space is so vast that these stars are just as big as Mother Earth, but they are so far away from us that they look like specks in the sky. The light you see from the stars is actually the reflection of the sunlight on them. It makes them look like they are shining from within but they are not.

"When I was just a boy," Kenny said, "my spirit used to travel into space where I would talk to my partners, these planets. It was just as plain as me here talking to you. If I had kept on trying to learn more about my medicine power for space, perhaps I could have done something important for my people. Instead, I got scared of my own medicine power.

"I never wanted to be any different from other people. So one day I just quit trying to learn about my medicine power. I act like I don't have any useful medicine power. I became a very quiet person. I don't talk much. I stay alone. I don't bother anyone at all. All my life I struggled to harvest food from the land just like everybody else. There were times when I was not fortunate to kill big game or catch fish. I became like a beggar and had to depend on others for food.

"All my life I wondered, 'Who is this man who came to me?' I can still see him dressed all in white. His hair is white and he looks very old. I think maybe he has some control over me that prevents me from telling for myself. He could be the Creator for all I know. Or perhaps he is a very high messenger for the Creator to have given me this power in an instant.

"I also wonder why I don't have more suitable medicine power that I could make use of to help myself and my people. But this old man gave me this medicine power. I didn't have any say in it. Maybe if I would have worked at it I could have found an important use for this power. But, I got scared instead.

"I suppose I could have taught people about the planets and space or somehow used the heat from the sun, or maybe I could have used the power to move or travel very fast. Who knows? All these things I may have done if I would have worked at it and tried, but I didn't.

"In the hand game," he said finally, "I took a small cone from the spruce tree that represented the moon spirit. This is what I saw the moon spirit do when he played hand games with the star spirits. I just copied what I saw them do." Then he laughed, "Those Yukon players had no idea what kind of medicine power I was using. You see, they don't have space medicine power. I've never heard of anyone else having it. If we had played a long time, we could have cleaned them out. But they saved themselves by quitting right away."

That is an account of the night Kenny explained about the stars, the sun, the moon, and Mother Earth to the Dene people.

12: Spirits and the Gift of Medicine Power

The stories of Edwar and Kenny were tales of men who received their medicine power before they were born. That means that the spirits of Edwar and Kenny received their medicine power from a very high guide and helper sent by the Creator.

Let me explain this. We believe that the Creator is responsible for creating all things, including all the spirits. Another name for spirit is "soul" or "ghost." Each person who is alive on Mother Earth today was once a spirit. When a child is born, their spirit is completely pure and very sacred and attached to their physical body. We do not believe that we are born with a mortal sin. We know that at birth we are completely sacred and pure. When the body dies, the spirit leaves the physical world and returns to the spirit world.

Most people cannot see spirits; however, some medicine people can see, hear, and communicate with spirits. Other medicine people have the ability to review the trail that a person's spirit has taken both in the past and into the future, as we learned in an earlier chapter. We call this power *Beh Gahley*. We know this because there have been some great medicine people who, over time, have shared their knowledge with the people. Animals also have a spirit and medicine power that they use to communicate with medicine people.

Some spirits are chosen by the Creator to receive medicine power before they are born into the physical world. The Creator has helpers or messengers that take care of this. The guide communicates with the spirit and says something like, "This is your medicine power. You own it all. Do the best you can and try to help others as much as possible." Then, that spirit becomes a medicine person when they are born into the physical world. The guide gives guidance and assistance to the person throughout his or her entire life. The guide doesn't tell the medicine person what to do. They only provide guidance. The medicine person

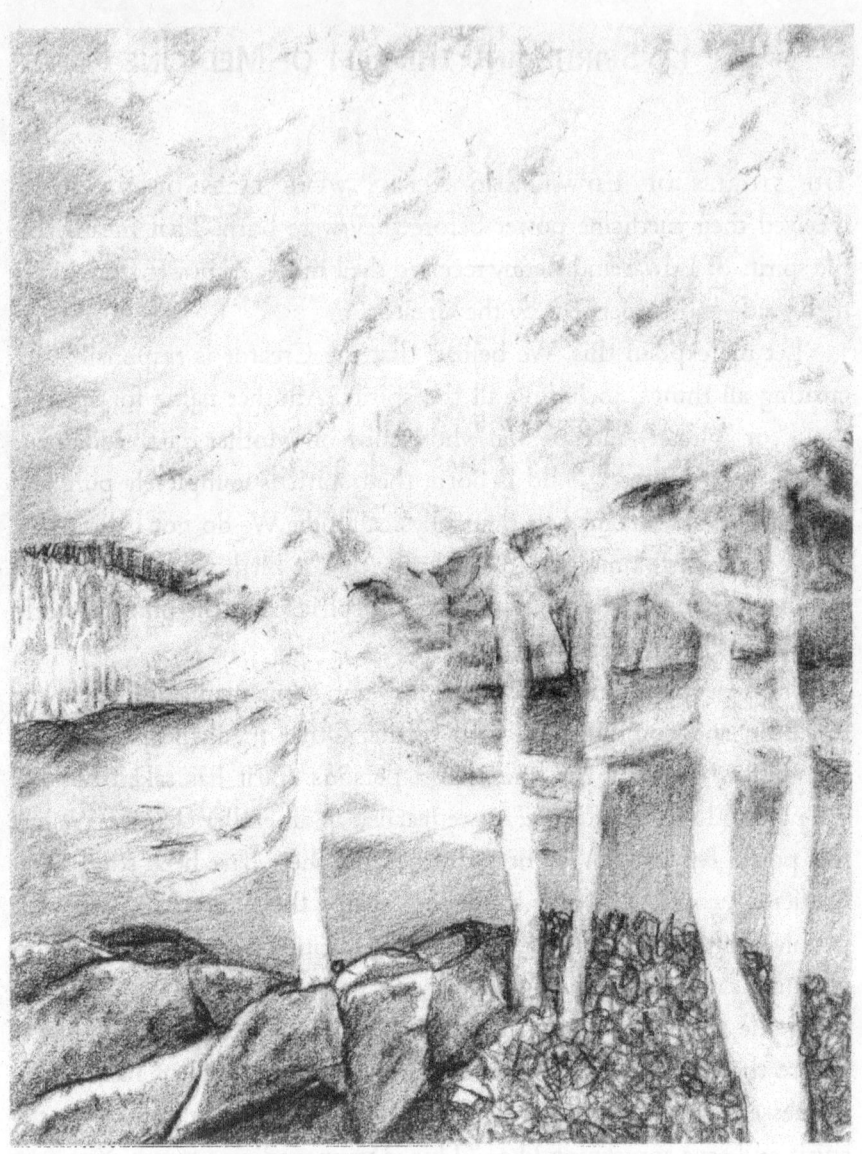

has the free will to decide how to conduct him or herself.

When the world was new, everyone wanted to be a medicine person, it seemed. Medicine power was highly valued; however, it was not easy to acquire. The Creator, in His infinite wisdom, knows who is fit for medicine power, even before that spirit is born into this physical world on Mother Earth. The Creator also makes all decisions regarding who will receive medicine power. Medicine power is sacred because it comes directly from the Creator. It is not an easy task to acquire medicine power if you are not born with it.

When the world was new, many people received medicine power before they were born, and they used their powers to help the people live. A medicine person needs to be intelligent and strong-willed to be able to discipline him or herself to use their medicine power for the right reasons. It is a grave responsibility to possess medicine power. Medicine power is intimately linked to the medicine person who owns it and responds to their feelings and intentions. This is why it is so important for a medicine person to stay in balance and in control of their thoughts, feelings, and actions. Whatever the medicine person does, the medicine power imitates.

Anger can easily lead to violent acts and even murder if a medicine person loses control. It is impossible to determine when someone is injured or killed through medicine power, unless another medicine person discovers the truth, as we will see in the stories that follow.

13: THE STORY OF PAUL BLONDIN

PAUL BLONDIN OF FORT NORMAN WAS A SECOND-CLASS MEDICINE man. Although he didn't have many different kinds of medicine power, what he did have was very powerful. He used his medicine power for the Eagle and mind control to help his people. He also had medicine power that made him a perfect shot with a rifle. He couldn't miss! Paul was a good man and well liked by the people for his generosity. He came from a big family, but, sadly, when he was a young man, his family was in a medicine-power conflict and many of his brothers and sisters died. This is that story.

His stepfather raised Paul because his own father died when he was young. His stepfather was a medicine man and a very quiet person. He rarely talked at all. Paul lived on the west end of Great Bear Lake, a place called Smith Arm. Dene always lived there because it is a place where people can fish all year round.

At this time, there was a strong but cruel medicine man living amongst them. People knew he owned a great deal of medicine power and were afraid of him. He was the worst kind of person. He would yell and take meat and fish away from others whenever he wanted. People believed he murdered with his medicine power but felt powerless to confront him or do anything about his behaviour.

Each summer, a group would paddle a small birch-bark canoe one hundred and twenty miles on the Great Bear Lake to reach the Barren lands. Here, they would hunt caribou and return with enough meat to last for a long time. It was a journey that took about six weeks to complete. This year, Paul was nineteen: young and strong, and among the group hunting for caribou.

The Elders of the group stayed behind at Smith Arm with some of the women and young children. They had been living at this one spot for months, catching many fish and drying most of them. The Elders complained that the camp was dirty and attracting too many flies, so they decided to move. They found an ideal spot not too far away and set up camp there.

It was a beautiful day. The lake was calm without a breeze in the air. Paul's stepfather searched and, after a time, found the perfect spot to set his fishnets. Just as he finished, he turned to find the hated medicine man behind him. The man bellowed, "What are you doing? I'm setting my nets here. Take your fish nets out of the water and move them!"

Paul's stepfather just looked at the man. He shook his head and said, "What is the matter with you? There is plenty of room on this huge

Great Bear Lake for many people to set their nets. Why do you want the spot where I have my nets?"

The evil medicine man screamed, "Maybe you don't want to live!"

Paul's stepfather answered, "Of course I want to live, just like anybody, but you are not going to push me around, old man!"

Then the evil man threatened, "You just talked yourself into an early grave. In two days you will be dead!" Paul's stepfather answered, "That's what you think! I have many years of life left in me."

The voices of the two angry men carried a long ways. The women on the shore heard everything and were very frightened. They knew that when a medicine person gets angry their medicine power is activated. Then their thoughts often become reality.

When the stepfather reached shore, the women ran to him and asked him, "Why are you quarrelling with that evil man? Now he will kill you, your wife, and all your family. Please go back to him with this gift we will give you and apologize. Do it before he goes to sleep tonight!"

But Paul's stepfather refused: "I will give him nothing. I am not scared to die. He has been treating people this way for too long now. Someone has to stand up to him!" Then he turned and went about his work as if nothing had happened.

Although it appeared that all was quiet in camp, it was not quiet in the medicine-power world. Immediately, the evil man went about making medicine power to attack Paul's stepfather, but he was surprised at what he found. The stepfather had medicine power to protect himself, and the evil man's assault was useless. He tried for three days but was unsuccessful. In frustration, he directed his efforts toward the stepfather's son, who died immediately. A great sorrow came upon the family.

When the stepfather used medicine to find out why the boy died, he discovered that the evil man had attacked the innocent child. He flew into a rage and lashed out with his medicine power to retaliate. Soon, the evil man's son was also dead.

At this time, Paul was hunting on the Barren lands, far away. He told his friend, "I don't feel right. I think something bad is happening, but I don't know what. I will have to make ceremony. Stay here and wait for me. I will go out alone to camp where I can have a ceremony in private. I will return when I know something. It won't be long."

Paul's strongest medicine power was for the Eagle, so he called the Eagle spirit to him. He asked, "Can you fly over the land and see what is happening?" Soon the Eagle spirit returned and said to him, "I have seen the trouble. A terrible conflict is happening with your family. Your stepfather and another man have been fighting with medicine power for days. They could not kill each other, so now they are killing each other's children. You are in grave danger. The man's medicine power will soon find you. You will need something to save you."

Then both Paul and the Eagle spirit held a ceremony. They were looking for some kind of medicine power that they could use to hide Paul from the danger that was coming. They had to find a kind of medicine power that Paul owned but that the evil man did not. Finally, they knew: the evil man did not have medicine power for the bottom of an Eagle nest. They decided that Paul would hide there for three days.

Before the ceremony was finished, Paul told the Eagle spirit, "I am glad we have found something to save my life, but still am I troubled. Can you check and see if my older sister is still alive?" The Eagle spirit soon told him, "She is."

"Good," Paul said, "then bring her spirit to me and I will hide it, too, at the bottom of the Eagle nest."

After three nights, Paul returned to the group that was hunting on the Barren lands. He told them, "Something terrible is happening to my family. I need to return as fast as possible." They left right away. Still, the journey was far, and it was storming and difficult to travel on the lake in their small birch-bark canoe. It was a long time before they finally reached their home camp.

Paul was unprepared for the great sorrow he found when he came upon his people. Paul learned that all five of his younger brothers and sisters were dead. The evil man's five children were also all dead. Of all the children in the two families, only Paul and his older sister were left alive. Paul was very angry because he knew for certain that all the deaths were a result of this medicine power conflict. He said, "Sister, I have returned with fat caribou meat. Cook it all. Then we will invite everyone to come and eat."

Soon, all were gathered for a great feast of caribou meat. Everyone was there except the evil man, so Paul went over to his tent. When he saw the pitiful old man grieving and alone, he felt a great anger about this terrible thing that was done. He grabbed the old man by his hair and walked him to the feast. He pushed him roughly to the ground. Paul's stepfather was right beside him.

Paul stood over the men and spoke in a loud voice: "Now that I have you both here there is something I want to say. You two men have killed ten innocent children with your dirty medicine power. What have you gained by this? Both of you are Elders and medicine men in our community. Everyone looks to you for guidance and protection. Instead, you have violated that trust and harmed our precious children. I am disgusted by your actions!"

Then Paul turned to the evil man and shouted, "It is your fault, old man. If you ever harm another person with medicine power, I will know and kill you myself. I could have done it but I let you live, even though you deserve to be burned alive for the crimes you have committed."

The two old men hung their heads in shame and cried to hear the truth spoken this way in public.

Paul continued, "I am the first person to ever talk to you this way, I know. And I see that you are crying for what you have done. When you return to the spirit world and have to face the Creator after what you have done here, then you will truly know the meaning of regret. That will be the time to cry." Then he faced the evil man once again, "I am warning you! Don't you ever harm another person again!"

Finally, he turned to the silent crowd and said to them, "I have finished what I had to say and you have all heard. Now it is time to move on. Please, everyone, let's eat."

From then on, the people had great respect for Paul because he had the courage to stand up to two strong medicine men. He was known for using medicine power to help people.

As the years passed, Paul married and had children of his own. Then one day he heard a woman crying loudly outside their tent. His wife rushed outside to see what was wrong and quickly returned to the tent. She said to him, "A young girl has a rabbit bone stuck in her throat and can't breathe. Her mother is trying to find someone to help her." Then she asked him, "Paul, years ago, before we were married, you told me you had medicine power to help when a person is choking. Were you just boasting or are you going to help this poor girl?"

With that, Paul burst out of the tent and let out a loud hoot. The bone shot out of the girl's mouth. Then he said, "What's the matter? We're supposed to be happy, but I hear crying. What's going on here?" The girl gasped for air and immediately recovered. Everyone nearby knew Paul had used medicine power to save the girl's life.

Another great story I'd like to share about Paul is about this one time he and his son Edward were hunting moose. It was getting dark and they had had no luck all day. Paul said, "We have to make camp and we'll find that moose tomorrow. It's a tricky one."

They had no food, just tea.

So they set up camp. They were growing hungrier by the second when here came a big Eagle. As you know, Paul had medicine power for the Eagle. He could talk to Eagles. Paul yelled at the Eagle and the Eagle took off and returned with a big trout, which it dropped by Paul's camp.

Boy, did they feast!

14: The Story of Bahwar and Yendee

Yendee and Bahwar were brothers. They were also two first-class medicine men from the Fort Wrigley area. They made history in this part of the country for their power in medicine. Several communities along the Mackenzie have access to the mountain ranges in the Yukon. These are places such as Fort Simpson, Fort Wrigley, Fort Norman, Fort Good Hope, Fort McPherson, and Aklavik. For many generations, the people from these areas survived by harvesting big game from the land.

Then, between 1870 and 1900, the gold rush brought many changes, including a mass of prospectors, Indian trappers and hunters, all travelling throughout the Northwest and Yukon territories. But more importantly, it brought something else that the Dene people were very interested in, as I mentioned before: the 30–30 repeating rifle.

Fur traders brought the rifles up the Pacific Coast in ships all the way from the United States. Then they sold them to the Dene people for a very high price. Still, the rifle was very useful to the Dene and was, therefore, a much sought after item. Many trappers from the Mackenzie River made the long journey into the Yukon just to purchase one of these rifles. This story is about five men from the Fort Wrigley area who did just that.

In 1890, Bahwar was a young man who had few fears, if any. The medicine power he possessed was very powerful and told him he would live to be an old man. Knowing this, he felt his life was secure. Perhaps this is why he acted in such reckless ways. Bahwar felt comfortable with strangers and relatives alike. He had medicine power to protect him and was therefore afraid of no one. It showed in his actions.

This was a time when the world was new. It was a time when Aboriginal people were thriving. Our numbers were great. Our medicine people were many. Life had an order to it as people followed Dene law and lived a traditional way of life.

Although there were many powerful medicine people, for the average person it was still difficult to know who they were. That is because, for the most part, medicine people do not talk about themselves and their power, especially to strangers. But Bahwar, like many other medicine-power people, had a special gift to tell when someone possessed medicine power. He could also tell when someone was using his or her medicine power.

One spring, he led five men into the Yukon Territory to purchase the precious 30-30 repeating rifles. They travelled a long way to reach their destination: a large village. The community consisted primarily of the Dene of the area, but there were many white prospectors as well. Not having travelled this way before, Bahwar didn't know anyone who lived in the village. Still, they knew of him. The tales of Bahwar, the medicine man from Fort Wrigley, had travelled far and wide, even reaching this village.

Now as it happened, Bahwar and his men arrived just as the village was preparing for a big feast and drum dance. As is customary, just prior to the food being served, the village leaders each took turns speaking to the crowd that had gathered. Then Bahwar himself stood up and addressed the people as a guest to their village. This is how most people were first introduced to Bahwar. When everyone had eaten all they could, a drum dance began.

When Dene people have a feast, much meat is eaten and this can cause people to tire easily once the drum dance starts. Often, one man will challenge another to see who will have the most stamina for dancing. It can start a friendly competition, and it seems there is always someone who shows off in this way.

This night, the drum dance was lively at first, but, as people got tired, fewer and fewer got up to dance. Seeing this, Bahwar called upon his animal dance medicine power to transform himself and his men. Then he yelled at them, "Get up and dance!" The men all danced in a lively way and seemed to gain energy the more they danced. First, as Bahwar

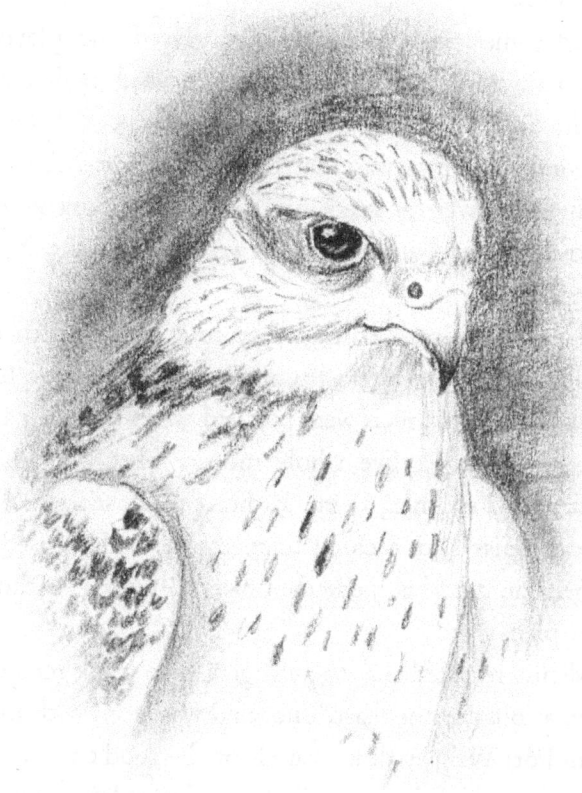

danced, he became as a bird, then a bear, then another animal, then a man again. He was shouting out to his men and laughing loud and long. The six men from Fort Wrigley danced every dance right to the end. All the people took notice, but they didn't like it. No one likes a stranger to come into their camp and beat them in such a proud way.

Bahwar didn't know if people realized he was using medicine power to dance, but he didn't care either. The more attention he got, the bolder he became. He was very daring.

The people from the village, offended by this arrogant and rude behaviour, decided to teach Bahwar a lesson. They challenged him and his men to a round of hand games. This time they were ready and planned to win at all costs.

The hand games were exciting. They played and played without stopping for two days and nights. Each side used medicine power to help them win. Still, no matter what the villagers did, Bahwar ultimately won each round. The fact was that Bahwar had medicine power that could literally overpower the medicine power his opponents were using. Bahwar was triumphant, but the villagers were growing angrier with these bigheaded strangers.

When the villagers realized that they could not beat them at hand games, they abruptly changed strategy and began to prepare a feast for the strangers. Bahwar and his men were puzzled when they saw the women getting prepared to cook five whole moose. This was an enormous amount of food for six men to eat. It didn't make sense. Bahwar knew something was amiss and decided to investigate. He sensed that they were in danger. He used his medicine power to read their thoughts and discover their plans.

The medicine revealed that the villagers were using medicine power in their preparations for the feast. The food was laced with medicine. If the men from Fort Wrigley didn't eat all of the food that was prepared, they would never make it home again. Even if they left now, they would never escape the medicine power released by this ceremony. Bahwar had to figure out a way to get rid of all the meat.

This time, he called on the monster medicine power to transform the men and himself. He took the men aside and told them, "We have much trouble here. Just do as I say and we'll be alright." Then he turned to the first man and told him quickly, "Open your mouth!" He carefully put something down his throat. "Now you will be able to eat a very great meal. We must eat all the food that they serve us or it will be our last meal." He turned to the other men and did the same.

When the feast was ready, the men sat down and ate and ate and ate. In a short time, all that was left was the broth the meat was cooked in. One man picked up the pot and drank that too. Eight pots of tea were placed before them. Each man grabbed a pot and poured it down his throat in one gulp. A group of people from the village was gathered near the strangers. They watched in disbelief and disgust to see men eat this way. Then, when all the food was gone, Bahwar stood up, stretched, smiled, and spoke in a loud voice to his men but so all could hear: "Well, that was good, but too bad these people have so little food to offer hungry strangers like us."

This enraged the villagers. A medicine war was on now.

Later that night a beautiful woman visited the men. She was striking, and the men noticed her right away. She smiled when she approached Bahwar and even he felt enchanted. She sat and talked with him, laughing and teasing and telling stories. Then she leaned near his ear and whispered, "Come sleep in my tent tonight."

Bahwar looked right into her eyes for a moment, then he nodded, and said, "Yes, I'll be there." The woman then quickly got up and left.

The other men were laughing and teasing Bahwar about the beautiful woman. But Bahwar wasn't laughing anymore. He'd never looked more serious. When Bahwar looked at that woman he could see more than just beauty. He could also see malice in her heart and evil intentions. He could see medicine power. He knew if he accepted her invitation he would die from the sickness she would give him. He also knew that the attraction all the men felt for her was a result of medicine power.

Still, later that evening, Bahwar took a walk to her tent. When he reached it, instead of going inside, he walked around the tent two times and then turned and returned to their camp. The next morning the woman was very sick. Her body swelled up and later she died.

When Bahwar awoke that morning, he told his men to get organized for the journey home. They had already traded for the rifles they wanted and all they had to do was pack up and they could be on their way.

The villagers had no intention of letting them get away that easily. A group of men approached Bahwar and said, "Let's play one more game before you leave. We will shoot targets. Whoever hits the most markers will win whatever is wagered. See these new 30–30 repeating rifles?"

Although they were anxious to go, Bahwar and his men could not think of a way out of playing this game. They said, "Fine, let's play one more game."

The village men said, "We will put a marker near that tree way over there. Why don't you and your men come and stand on this side and we will shoot first?" However, they were not fooling Bahwar. All this time, Bahwar was reading their minds and saw that they had no intention of shooting the markers. They intended to shoot Bahwar and his companions. The villagers prepared themselves as if to shoot the markers and then turned suddenly to face Bahwar and his men.

Just then, Bahwar shouted out in a loud and powerful voice. Right before their eyes, the barrels of the guns melted and dripped to the ground. A heap of melted steel lay on the ground. Bahwar walked over to the mound, bent over, and, with his bare hands, gathered up the metal. He moulded it briefly and then shot the marker to pieces.

The villagers backed away in terror. Then Bahwar turned to them and said, "What's the matter? Why don't you shoot the marker? As you can see, I have no problem hitting it. But then again, you may have a problem. If we start a war here, your guns are going to be all melted down on the ground. But mine is fine." Then in a rage, he roared, "In fact, you're lucky I don't shoot you all right here, right now!"

Then he called to his men, "Let's get out of here."

They grabbed their rifles and packs and started off into the mountains as quick as they could go. Their journey was going to be a long one. It was four hundred miles to Fort Wrigley. They ran as far as they could; then they walked.

As Bahwar walked, he summoned medicine power to discover what the villagers did once they had left. He saw that they were more furious than ever and were certainly not going to let Bahwar and his men walk away unharmed. Instead, they planned to hunt Bahwar down and kill him and his men.

Bahwar thought carefully. It was still his responsibility to get the men home safely. "Let's make a camp here," he said, "but only for a short while. There is something I must do." The men were grateful for the rest and lay down to sleep.

Then Bahwar went straight to his work. He gathered together his sacred things, then sat on the ground. Bahwar closed his eyes and began to sing a very sacred song. After a time, the men awoke. Bahwar was still sitting on the ground, eyes closed. He seemed to be talking to someone, but the men could only hear him mumble. They knew he was calling on medicine power.

The men were hungry and quickly fixed themselves some food before Bahwar had a chance to announce it was time to leave. Suddenly, Bahwar spoke to them: "Come here. I will do something to help us all, but you must follow exactly what I say. I am going to summon medicine power that will make it easier for each of you to make the long journey home at a very quick pace."

He took out some doctor medicine and told each man, "Rub this all over your face." While they worked with the medicine, Bahwar closed his eyes and mumbled in a soft voice. Then he told them, "This medicine power will keep you from feeling hungry on our journey home." Then he ordered, "Remove your pants and rub this medicine on your legs. This medicine will keep you from getting tired on the journey home."

Then, while they worked with the medicine again, he closed his eyes and mumbled in a soft voice. Finally he said, "Put this medicine in your eyes. It will keep you from getting sleepy on our long journey home."

When the ceremony was finished, the men broke camp and started off. After a time they came upon the biggest river in the north: the Mackenzie River. Without stopping, Bahwar reached into the river, grabbed a handful of sand, and threw it into the water. Then he stepped right into the river on top of the sand he had just tossed. Suddenly, it had become very shallow there. The men followed right behind him and crossed the entire river that way, walking across it as if it were a shallow creek. Within two nights they had travelled the four hundred miles and were approaching their own community.

Before they reached home, Bahwar stopped to speak to his men: "When our relatives ask about our trip we will tell them that we had fun and it was a good journey. We won't ever tell anyone about the troubles we've been through or how medicine power helped us. Something serious could happen. Do you understand?" The men agreed. They all knew Bahwar wouldn't want his brother, Yendee, to know anything about what had happened.

Bahwar hoped their troubles were far behind, but medicine power is a spirit and very powerful. Distance is nothing to a Spirit; it can follow you no matter where you go.

In the fall, the people of Fort Wrigley worked hard to harvest the land for winter. The Mackenzie River is not a good river for fish, so the people travelled inland to hunt moose, woodland caribou, and snare rabbits. There was a smaller river not too far away that the people liked for fishing. There, the women gathered brush for the tepees and wood for the fires.

Dene people have a history of conflicts with other tribes. There are a number of different nations in the north, and, for the most part, they don't get along very well. One difficulty we've had is that we speak different languages. Even amongst the Dene tribes there is a number of different dialects: North and South Slavey, Dogrib, Gwich'in, and Chipewyan.

Then there are other nations besides the Dene as well. For some reason we've all probably forgotten, we don't mix with each other very much. It's as if we are complete strangers. Something else that has caused many problems is the use of medicine power against people and other tribes.

Generally, people have great respect for medicine power, even though they often don't really understand it. The average person—someone without medicine power—will only learn how it works through the teachings of Elders.

When the world was new, it was common for Elders to meet each day in a public gathering place and teach about many things, even medicine power. Most people do not have personal experience with medicine power, so they have to trust the Elders' teachings. The best they can do is to follow Dene laws that teach how to live with each other peacefully and to adhere very closely to the medicine-power laws that are taught by the Elders. Besides, everyone has heard the storytellers tell the many tales of people who used their medicine power to harm others. This instills fear in many and further motivates people to follow the strict teachings of medicine-power law and try to get along with everyone.

In Fort Wrigley, disturbing news was spreading that someone had heard whistling while they were hunting alone out in the bush. Then someone else said that "bushmen" had pulled all their fish nets out of the water, and someone else was convinced that the "bushmen" damaged all their rabbit snares. The fear was contagious, and soon people were afraid to leave their camp. The men weren't hunting, and the people were running out of food.

The Elders met and decided to approach the two strongest medicine men they had: Vendee and Bahwar. They pleaded with them: "The children are hungry. Everyone is afraid to go out on the land to hunt. Can you do something?"

Vendee and Bahwar listened closely. Then Vendee spoke up, "Why would a small problem like a bushman cause so much trouble for my people? I can't stand to see you all suffer like this. I will do what I can." Then he said, "Bring me a moose hide and spread it on the ground right here. Then make a big fire beside it."

Vendee closed his eyes and started to sing a song. When he was finished he spoke so quietly no one could quite hear his words. The people watched intently. Then, very faintly, the crying of children and adults could be heard. The crowd strained to see and hear. The sound grew louder until everyone was sure. The cries were coming from the moose hide. Vendee stood up and took the moose hide in his hands. As soon as his fingers touched the hide, the eerie sound grew. Vendee continued with his soft-spoken words. Then, without warning, he threw the hide on the fire. A great tower of fire erupted on the spot. Vendee continued to sing until the hide had been reduced to ashes.

He turned to the crowd and said, "It is done! I have killed all the Bushmen spirits, whoever they were. They are all dead now. You are safe to go back hunting and travelling in the bush all you want."

And they did. Life continued as it had before. Groups went out fishing. Others went out hunting. The fear was gone. But the Elders talked among themselves and they were not pleased. They said, "It is never good to kill many people all at once, like what has just happened here. Whoever was killed by Vendee's medicine power will have relatives somewhere who will be affected by this. They will be very angry. This could cause us much trouble."

An Elder who was sitting in the back listening to all the talk finally spoke up. He said, "I have been thinking about this for a long time and I wonder if what we have here is a medicine war. I also wonder if it has something to do with Bahwar's trip to the Yukon Territory. If it is, we have not seen the end of our troubles yet."

Soon afterward, the wise Elder's words came true. A sickness spread throughout the community. Many people fell ill and soon died. Even the medicine people were dying. It was pitiful. The people were too sick to hunt and fish and soon they were starving.

A group of Elders ordered, "Have the men who made the trip to the Yukon come to us now!" Soon these men were sitting in front of them with very solemn faces. One Elder came right to the point: "You have told us that your trip to the Yukon went very well. You say you had a peaceful visit with the people there. I do not believe this anymore. I believe you have caused these problems we are all having now. Are you ready to lose your wives and other family members? That is what is happening. For the good of your people, you must tell us the truth about what happened on your journey. Maybe then we will be able to save ourselves."

After hearing this, the men told the Elders the real story about the Yukon journey.

The Elders approached Bahwar and Vendee and asked them to use their medicine power to discover what was causing the sickness among the people. Bahwar was quiet. He already knew what had caused the trouble. He had seen it. But Vendee wanted to help the Elders and his people and went ahead with preparations.

Vendee conducted a medicine ceremony. He sang many songs and, eyes shut, mumbled many quiet words talking to the spirits. When he was finally finished he turned to his people with a pained look on his face and told them, "I have very bad news to tell you today. A terrible mistake has happened here. We have killed our own people. The Bushmen spirits that were killed when I made medicine were actually not Bushmen at all. They are us, our own people. I have seen it. It is so. Only a few will survive."

Then he took a deep breath and deadly rage filled his face. He bellowed, "My brother! He is a fool! It is his fault! If he had told us what he did when he was in the Yukon we would not be in this trouble now." Then he looked away as if he was seeing far into the distance. Vendee declared, "But those people who have sent us this sickness will also pay for their foolishness. I have sent the sickness back to them. They will know what it is to lose so many relatives in a medicine war." Of the many stories about medicine power, this is the cruelest story told about the work of medicine power.

DEFINING MEDICINE POWER

One of the medicine-power laws teaches, "Be careful in all you do to avoid injuring the feelings of others." Everyone is taught medicine-power laws. Elders teach these laws to their people and tell the stories of what happens when the laws are not followed. Still, for someone who is not a medicine person, it can be hard to understand or even believe the teachings about medicine power. It is something that requires faith until you have the experience yourself. Then you realize why the medicine-power laws have been established and why it's so important that everyone follow them.

Medicine-power law teaches us to avoid hurting the feelings of others, arguing, and fighting. You are advised to try to please others. When you live by these laws, you are truly a good citizen of the community and are respected for it. If Bahwar had respected this law, he would have travelled to the Yukon community, bought his guns, and then gone home quietly. But he was a young man: proud and reckless, and showing off was too big a temptation for him to resist.

It is not unusual for a medicine person to recognize another medicine person, even the first time they meet. If they have medicine power for the same item, they may know each other in the spirit world long before they ever meet in the physical world. It is possible that a medicine person from the Yukon village recognized Bahwar from the spirit world even though they were meeting for the first time in their village. He or she may have known Bahwar was a medicine person and the powers he possessed.

It is considered a great offence, in the eyes of medicine people, to show off and take advantage of others through the use of your medicine power. Bahwar did this in many different ways. First, Bahwar's proud display of dancing all night without tiring was such an offence. People say Bahwar used animal dancing power to transform into a bird. These birds, a kind of chicken, are known to dance in the springtime, sometimes for days at a time. Bahwar used the chicken spirit to dance and dance without tiring.

Second, when Bahwar played hand games, he used his medicine power to read the minds of his opponents. This way he could learn in which hand they put the object they were trying to hide. That's how he won the game.

Third, Bahwar used his power to read minds to learn what the beautiful woman who came to him was planning. She was sent by others to get rid of Bahwar. But, in revenge, he used his power over the human body to slow her heart down until it finally stopped, killing her.

Fourth, Bahwar used power over the elements to melt the barrels of the rifles. The way this works is very fascinating. In the beginning of time, before the creation of Mother Earth, a part of the sun broke away and began to float in space, still immensely hot. This part is what we now call a planet. On this piece existed every kind of element and mineral that we know about. One of those minerals was metal; only, at that time, the planet was so hot that it was a liquid.

There have been several powerful medicine-power people who possess this power that comes from the beginning of time. Melting metal in an instant is easy for a medicine person with this power, such as Bahwar was. Still, how he shot the gun after it was melted into a heap is a true mystery.

It is likely that the medicine people from the Yukon village were also very strong. When they competed with Bahwar in a direct way they lost. Therefore, they knew that if they were going to beat him it would have to be through trickery. At first, when Bahwar and his men fled home, the Yukon people tried to follow them, but after only a short ways, they gave up. Still, they were determined to retaliate. They came up with a plan to use medicine power to trick Bahwar.

The Yukon medicine people transformed the spirits of the people of Fort Wrigley into the spirits of Bushmen. Then, when Vendee attempted to rid the area of the Bushmen spirits that his people were so afraid of, he mistakenly attacked the spirits of his own people. If he had taken the time to investigate before he decided on an action, he would have realized this. After he discovered his mistake, it was too late. Many people died. In retaliation, Vendee sent the sickness back to the Yukon people and many people died there. This is the cost of a medicine-power war.

15: The Story of Ehdah

EHDAH WAS A MEDICINE MAN FROM FORT GOOD HOPE, NWT. He was a *Beh Bah Teh*, which, when translated into English, actually means "a person with medicine power that is far greater than others." There are many stories about the *Beh Bah Teh* of the past because they have done wondrous things that fascinate people. Ehdah was one of them.

Ehdah told his people, "Every day, since the time I was just a baby, I have been visited by vision power, my spirit teacher." Similar to children that attend school each day, Ehdah was being taught important lessons about medicine power that he would need in his life. This is how medicine people gain knowledge of the spirit world that other people do not have.

Ehdah lived most of his life in two communities: Fort Good Hope and Arctic Red River, NWT. It is two hundred miles between these two settlements. Ehdah spent his summers on the Mackenzie River fishing. It is still common for people of the area to work hard to catch and dry all the fish they can in the summer. In winter there is not one fish in the river.

When they harvest fish they save the fish guts. For storage they put the fish guts in a birch-bark container, dig a hole in the ground, and place the container up against the permafrost. This way the flies don't get at it and it remains cool. They feed dry fish and fish guts to their dogs. That is the way people of the area survive.

Ehdah spent time on the east side of the river, which is a huge, mountainous area toward the Yukon border. Ehdah was a Mountain Dene as well. He was a very strong medicine-power person, and many people didn't like him but felt safer living close to him. He attracted many people to him. Ehdah usually lived with a large group of people wherever his travels took him.

Sometimes when a medicine person begins to help others with

medicine power, he or she attracts unwanted attention from other medicine people. It may even lead to an attack on the person. He or she must resort to acts of protection and self-defense. It can become a very dangerous situation when a medicine person fights back against an attack with medicine power.

This is what we call a medicine-power conflict, or war. It can become so serious that one of the opponents can lose his or her life in the conflict. However, even a death doesn't guarantee the conflict will end. Relatives of the deceased person may decide to retaliate in revenge. This creates a bigger problem that can last for a long time.

Ehdah experienced this in his life. It seemed people would not leave him alone. Ehdah lived with a large group of people in the mountain region. The Fort Norman Mountain people and the Tutchone tribe from Fort McPherson frequented that area as well. In the winter, they all utilized the resources of this area and would naturally encounter each other from time to time.

It is rare for a *Bah Beh Teh* to be shy or afraid of others because they can be assured of the protection of strong medicine. This was true of Ehdah. He spoke freely even to strangers, for he feared no one.

The Tutchone tribe knew Ehdah well. They recognized him as a strong medicine man and the leader of a large group of people. One winter, the Tutchone suffered greatly. In spite of their efforts, they were unable to harvest big game from the mountain region. This was perilous because there were no fish in the rivers at that time of year and the people depended on hunting to survive.

By the middle of the winter, the Tutchone people were running out of food. They faced starvation. First the dogs began to die, then the people. The group walked, pulling their small toboggans, in search of others who could help them. Although they helped each other and shared what they had, many still perished. Medicine people attempted to use medicine power to hunt but were unsuccessful.

In search of an explanation for the tragic circumstances they found themselves in, one Tutchone medicine man accused Ehdah of using medicine to make the animals disappear in their area. He said that Ehdah was responsible for the suffering the people endured and the death of those who had starved.

The people talked and talked about his claim against Ehdah. Many Tutchone, especially those who had lost loved ones, were very angry. They decided to band together to get rid of Ehdah by using medicine power. When spring finally arrived, they travelled to their fish camp to make dry fish. Other groups of Tutchone gathered here also, and together they went about making medicine to get rid of Ehdah.

The Tutchone people did not intend to walk over to Ehdah and confront him directly. Instead, they planned to use the medicine-power spirits. Four strong medicine-power spirits of the Tutchone people would go to Ehdah, wherever he was fishing, and get rid of him with medicine power. That was the plan.

Ehdah was at a fish camp making dry fish with his people. One day, after checking his nets, he returned to camp with a canoe full of fish. Just as he reached the shore, he took one step out of the kayak, leaned on his paddle, and suddenly fell to the ground, clutching his chest. People began screaming, "Ehdah has fallen to the ground!"

They quickly wrapped him in a tarp and carried him to his tent. Group members who possessed medicine power were summoned to help him. They sang to make medicine over him and to find out what happened. Nothing seemed to help. One Elder yelled at Ehdah, "We can't find out what the problem is with you. You will have to help yourself." Ehdah said, "Yes, have the young boys run into the bush. I want a chicken right now." Parents told their sons to go hunting for chickens and bring them back as quickly as possible.

Soon after, one boy brought them two chickens. Ehdah told his wife to open the ribs of the chicken and cut out the heart. He then said, "Give it to me." So his wife removed the heart and gave it to her husband. Ehdah held the small chicken heart in the palm of his hand

and struggled to pronounce a strange wording. He mumbled briefly and then said, "Creator, I beg you to transform the chicken heart into mine to restore my life."

With these words he pressed the chicken heart into his chest. A minute later he pulled his hand away and the heart was gone. He mumbled to himself briefly and then turned to those watching and said, "I'm okay now. I will live with this chicken heart for the rest of my life. There is no more need to worry about me. But now, I will make medicine power to discover what has happened to me."

For an hour he sang and mumbled to the medicine-power spirits. Then he explained to the people: "A Tutchone tribe did this to me. Last year the people suffered a terrible winter where many perished from starvation. They blame their misfortune on me. They have tried to kill me with their medicine power and they were almost successful, but I have stopped them. Now they will have to pay. I will wait until winter comes again."

In November of the next year the people were once again in mountain country. Ehdah summoned a north wind to blow on Tutchone country. It continued for many weeks. The country was so cold that hunting was impossible and the people faced starvation once again. Many dogs perished and, tragically, more people died, too.

Throughout the winter, they came together to make medicine to help themselves. But nothing changed. Ehdah overpowered their medicine with his own resources. The Tutchone people struggled until spring arrived. By spring, they were resigned to make peace with Ehdah.

Thirty canoes travelled to Fort Good Hope to see Ehdah. An Elder, who was selected to represent the group, went up to Ehdah and spoke directly to him: "We have come here to make peace with you. It's no good to hate each other. Besides, it is not our way to hate. If we keep on this way, many will die."

The Tutchone's Elder pleaded with Ehdah, "I ask you to accept our offer. We have brought many gifts for you."

Ehdah replied, "I accept your offer of peace. The Creator has given us medicine power to do good deeds, to share, and to help everyone we can. Still, we push each other around and start conflicts with our medicine power. People have lost their lives. It is wrong, I agree. It is the wrong attitude for us to have. We have created problems for ourselves. I hope the Creator will forgive us for the mistakes we have made here. We will pray and ask for forgiveness. I agree with you that peace between us is better. We will not do that again. Let us help the people instead with our gifts of medicine power."

With that, peace was established between the two tribes. The Tutchones presented many gifts to Ehdah. They offered a new birch-bark canoe, a moose-hide jacket, a sheep-hide jacket, blankets, rugs, moccasins, spears, a bow and arrow, and even a tent. It was a great day, and, to honour the occasion, a feast was prepared, followed by two days of drum dancing. This was a historic and monumental event for northern Aboriginal people.

When the world was new, these kinds of things happened often. A medicine-power conflict can start a big war throughout the country. This is the way the problem with Ehdah started. Ehdah's story illustrates the strength of some medicine power. One person, Ehdah, was able to overpower the whole Tutchone tribe with his medicine power. No one could do anything to him and he knew that he could overpower everyone. So, when the world was new, a person like Ehdah could do a lot of damage with a violent action. Even just one man could cause great harm if he felt pushed to act.

Of the many kinds of medicine power, there is one called sacred medicine power. This refers to when a medicine person counsels the people about the Creator's teachings. In fact, the medicine-power person communicates with this sacred power, or sacred spirit. That is why they teach about the Creator.

Yamoria, Ehtseo Ayah, and Ehdah all communicated with the sacred medicine power, which is what motivated them to devote their lives to helping their people as much as they could.

16: Lost!

MEDICINE POWER HAS EXISTED FOR A VERY LONG PERIOD OF TIME. How do we know this? Dene people have a strong tradition of storytelling. This is how we passed on our history to new generations. Whenever there was a gathering of people, Elders would tell stories. Still, today, people love to hear medicine stories and storytellers love to tell them. The more unusual or miraculous the event, the more often the story is told. This next story is about a Dogrib man who was lost and the efforts made with medicine power to find him.

In the year 1900, Dene people were still surviving by harvesting food from the land and trapping for furs to trade with the fur traders. The Dogrib people of the Fort Rae area travelled a great deal searching for food. They would come to the fort for a few days but then return to the bush to hunt and trap.

The Dogrib people traded caribou hides, strip string for snowshoes, dry meat, bone grease, and pounded meat. They travelled to the Barren lands to hunt caribou in the fall and store food for winter. The Dogrib territory was very big in those days, and there were many different routes to travel to the Barren lands.

In this story, a group of ten families set off one summer walking with packs to the Barren lands. They followed the timberline, stopping regularly for a day or two to hunt for moose and woodland caribou. One day, a man set off for the day to hunt moose. When he did not return by night, the group thought he must have camped where he was. But by the second night they became alarmed. They set off the next morning to look for him, but even after searching for two days, they could not find him.

There were two medicine men within the group who made a ceremony to investigate what happened to the man, but they discovered nothing. So the group sent out a runner to find a group of Dogrib people who had taken a different route to the Barren lands. Among this group was a medicine man that they hoped could help them. They needed help from someone who had medicine power to see *Beh Gahley*, the Trail of the Spirit.

They were very relieved to see their runner and the medicine man

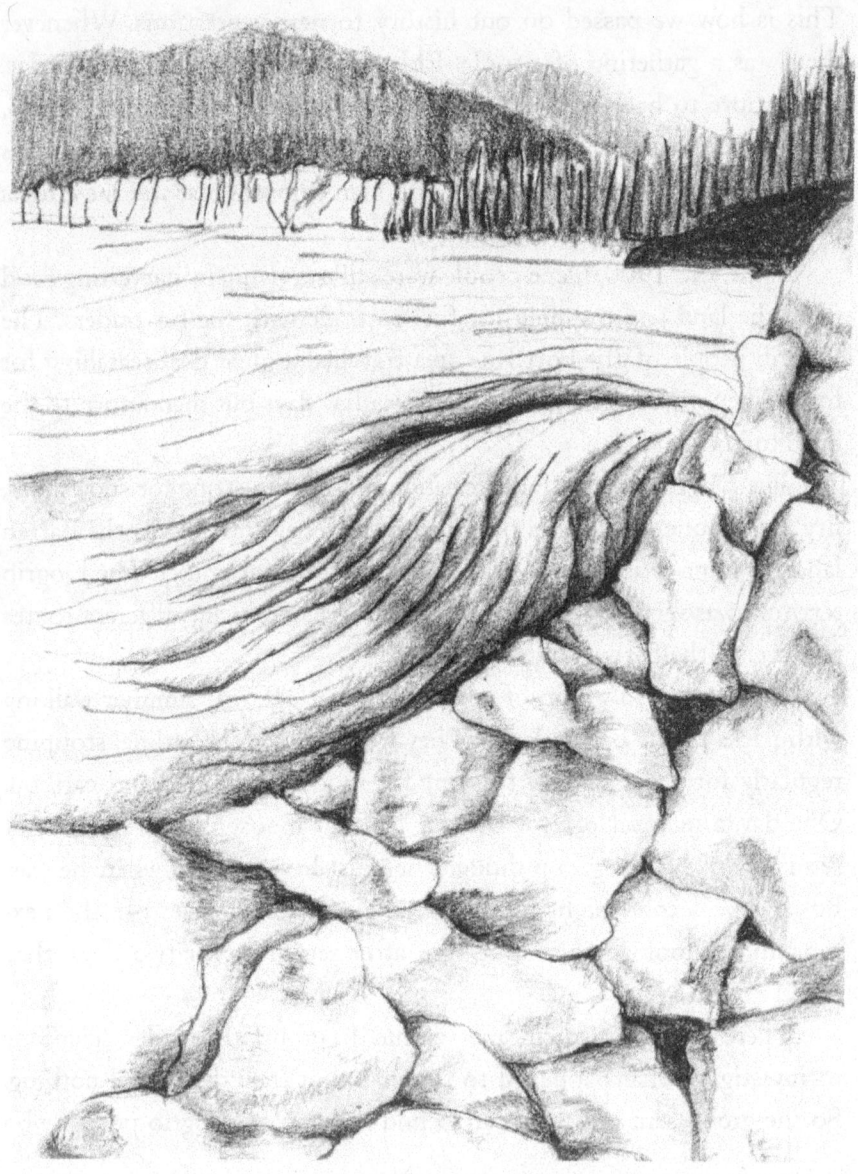

return to their camp. They quickly fed them and made the medicine man comfortable. Then he began a ceremony to trace the lost man's *Beh Gahley*. After a long while, the medicine man sat back and appeared to be thinking very seriously. Then, abruptly, he said, "I will try again!"

Again he went through the ceremony. Finally, he turned to the people to speak: "My friends and relatives, my medicine power is limited. Some people are very lucky to have medicine power that takes the form of a human person and will actually show a medicine person where someone or something is. But, this is not true for me. As you probably know, I have medicine power for *Beh Gahley*. I have tracked the trail of this man's spirit from the time he began walking away from your group. And, I must say, I have retraced it twice to be sure. This is what I saw.

"There is a narrow lake facing north about a two-hour walk from here. There is a rocky ridge on the far side of the lakeshore. One part is very steep right down into the lake. I traced the spirit to that rock ridge where the steep bank goes into the lake. But I did not see him there. Sometimes, when a person's body dies, his spirit will stay close by for a long time. Other times, the spirit leaves right away. In this case, there is nothing for me to see. Therefore, I'm sorry to say that I think your relative is dead. I feel sure that his body is on the far side of the lake where the bank is steep and there is a rock ridge. That is why his spirit's trail ends there. I suggest you send people to find him right away."

Sadly, when the group made a thorough search of the spot that the medicine man had described, they found the lost hunter, dead. This story shows how important medicine power was to our people at that time.

17: Dene Prayer

Aboriginal people all over the world have always had great devotion to the Creator. Dene people have our own way of prayer. We have learned these ways from teachings that have been given to us for generations by many prophets and holy persons who lived among our people. Dene people use the word "Creator," rather than the word "God" like the Europeans, because it is closer to the translation from our languages. *Ne Wesiene* is literally translated to "the Creator of all land."

Also, we know that prophets are sent here by the Creator to teach us how to live a better way of life. It is said that, long ago, Dene life was very difficult and that the people did not live like human beings. We did not work collectively to get things done and, therefore, survival was precarious. The Creator saw the Dene people struggling and took pity on us. He arranged for Yamoria, the prophet, to come to the people and teach us a better way of life. Yamoria is responsible for establishing Dene laws. Sometimes he is called "The Great Lawmaker." He taught us a way of life that promotes co-operation, sharing, and living in harmony with one another.

Prophets are created the same way as first-class medicine people. Even before the person is born, the Creator chooses him or her to fulfill this role in life. The prophet has a vision in which one of the Creator's helpers or messengers comes to him or her and presents them with the knowledge they need to become teachers of the people. Of course, regardless of how much knowledge or medicine power they are given, it is transferred to them in an instant. We are reminded that nothing is impossible for the Creator.

It is important to know that, to the Dene, all things created by the Creator also represent the Creator and are very sacred. We have been taught by hundreds—or perhaps even thousands—of different Elders over the generations about how to pray to the Creator. This is why there are so many different ways for us to pray. We have been told to ask for help to survive in our lands.

We have also been told that the sun, moon, stars, mountains, big lakes, and all things in creation are representatives of the Creator, and, therefore, it is wise to ask these creations for help whenever you approach them. When Dene people travel and come upon one of these landmarks, we will stop and pray and make little offerings of whatever we have to the lake or mountain or other representative.

Another way that we pray is through sacred prayer songs and drum songs. These songs usually come to us through a vision. The prophets have taught us the prayer and drum songs over time and there are quite a few now. It was common for people to travel very far to hear a prophet teach and to learn their prayer songs. Aboriginal people love and respect our way of life that honours these prayer songs.

As you may know, the missionaries tried to stop us from singing our songs, thinking that, somehow, they were evil. Of course, we could never do that and so, fortunately, we still have many traditional songs. When the Pope visited some years ago, he asked the Dene people to try to forgive the missionaries for the way they treated our people. This was very good. Since then, it is more common for Dene people to sing our prayer and drum songs in the church.

When the first Europeans came to the north they thought they were the master race of the world. Their culture already included the Industrial Revolution, while we were still harvesting the land to survive. They thought we were inferior and they seemed to hate us. They called us names such as "savages" and "pagans." Naturally, this was a grave mistake and was the basis of many unjust things that have happened to our people. They did not understand that the Dene, who met those first Europeans years and years ago, were praying to the same God that the prophet Moses prayed to, as told in the Bible.

Sometimes I think it's no wonder that the Europeans didn't like us. They likely had never seen people singing, yelling, and dancing the way we do, or praying to each of these great creations of the Creator. But, try as they might, they could not get rid of us. We are a tough people and we are still here.

18: THE WAY OF PROPHETS AND MIRACLES

WHEN THE WORLD WAS NEW, THERE WERE MANY PROPHETS. THE Creator gave prophets the ability to create miracles to help the people believe that what they were saying was true. The powers that are given to prophets are not the same as other medicine powers. Dene prophets receive what we call "Holy Medicine Power."

The prophets' role is to teach the people that the Creator exists and how to live a good life here on Mother Earth. Some Dene prophets had the power to predict what was going to happen in the future. This kind of power is highly respected. Most prophets receive holy medicine power before they are born, but some receive it later.

One Dene prophet who received holy medicine power after he was born, was Ehtseo Ayha of Déline, who died in 1940. He received a visit from one of the Creator's helpers and messengers when he was a teenager. He was told that the messenger would return someday to gift him with holy medicine power. "In the meantime, live as good a life as you can," the messenger told him. Ayha told the messenger that he expected the helper to return right away. In truth, it was forty years before he was visited. Then he was given the knowledge of what he was to teach to the people.

Prophets were also known for bringing prayer and drum songs to the people. One such person was a mountain Dene from Fort Norman, NWT. In one year, he received fifty-two prayer songs. Twenty of those songs are still sung today. Other prophets had other prayer songs. Even today, when a feast is about to begin, Elders take out their drums and sing some of these sacred songs.

Of course, no chapter about prophets would be complete without mentioning Yamoria, The Great Lawmaker. He was a great medicine man and had a vast knowledge of how medicine power worked. In the years before Yamoria came to my people, there was great chaos. There were many medicine people who misused their sacred gifts from the Creator. Murder with medicine power was rampant. Many medicine people treated others in a very bad way.

Yamoria could not tolerate this kind of behaviour and spent his life travelling all over the north. Wherever groups of people would gather, he would be there pleading with the people to change their behaviour and help each other with medicine power. He encouraged the people to appoint a strong medicine person to be their leader who could then help to organize the people to work together. Yamoria advised, "Don't ever use medicine power to hurt another person!"

One day he faced two medicine people who were very angry and threatened by what he was teaching. Together they challenged Yamoria and tried to intimidate him. Yamoria knew that these men were two of the worst offenders of using medicine power to harm others. A great argument ensued. The two men were yelling at Yamoria and threatening him. Then, just as the confrontation began to escalate, Yamoria clapped his hands and the two men crumpled to the ground in a heap. They were dead. A large crowd that witnessed the event stood in shocked silence.

Yamoria warned the crowd, "From this day forward, if any of you use medicine power to harm others, I will know. Even if I am travelling far away from here, I will see whatever you do. Those who continue to harm others do not deserve to live with the rest of these good people. And I will make sure you do not live anymore!"

The people were scared.

He instructed the people to hold a gathering at the end of each day when the work was done. Then he entrusted the Elders with a grave responsibility. He taught, "At the end of the day, when the work is done, meet in the gathering place. Here the Elders will give you a valuable gift: the teachings of how to live a good life with medicine power. They will share the stories of all the good things that have happened when medicine power is used right and all the terrible things that have happened when it is used wrong. The gathering place is for everyone young and old. You can bring the children as soon as they can talk. Even in the day, bring the children to the gathering place and let the Elders teach the children the things they need to know to grow up to be good people.

"I am going to give you some medicine-power laws for everyone to follow. It is the role of the Elders to make sure everyone knows about these laws and understands them. When they are followed, life will be very good for everyone. It's important that you do this everyday so you can govern yourself and work hard together from now on."

It was true. Dene people established this tradition of gathering together every night to tell stories and teach about Dene law and how to become good people, and life became much better for us. This is also how history was preserved. The events of the past have been told and retold hundreds—maybe thousands—of times over the generations. We even have stories about the dinosaurs.

19: The Challenges of Living with Medicine Power

POSSESSING MEDICINE POWER REQUIRES GREAT SELF-DISCIPLINE because there are rules that each medicine person must follow. The medicine person is actually in partnership with the medicine-power spirit and, like other relationships, the medicine person must be aware of things that the medicine-power spirit doesn't like. Then there are specific things that they must do and other things that they must not do.

It's possible to be in conflict with your own medicine power because you have not followed the rules and guidelines set down for you. It's also possible for the medicine power to leave you. Medicine power is only on loan. When the medicine person's body dies, and they return to the spirit world, their medicine power leaves them and returns to the Creator. Later, the Creator may choose to loan the medicine-power spirit to another person when they are born into the physical world. The medicine-power spirit has a life of its own and it never dies. This is why a medicine person does not have complete control of their medicine power.

Another challenge for medicine people is the dual lives that they must live. On the one hand, they live a life similar to the life of someone who is not a medicine person. But, on the other hand, and, at the same time, they live the life of a medicine person who has a spirit partner. They must follow certain rules or get into trouble, and much of this second life can never be spoken about to anyone.

Still, a medicine person has special gifts to be used to help their people. It is common for a whole community to rely on their medicine people. Requests for help can be many, and the medicine person's life is not their own. The stronger the person's medicine power, the more people will come wanting help. A medicine person can sometimes be faced with an onslaught of requests for help and must possess endless generosity and selflessness to endure.

Some of the rules regarding medicine power even apply to people who do not possess medicine power. For example, each person must have good thoughts, respectful of all people and animals. People have found themselves in trouble even for thinking wicked thoughts. Let me explain.

Suppose an individual had lustful thoughts about another person, but that person just happens to be a strong medicine person who can control minds and read thoughts. The medicine person would know about the lustful thoughts and may attack the offender. There are many stories about people getting murdered with medicine power for thinking wicked thoughts about a medicine person.

When the world was new, and there were many, many powerful medicine people, unlike today when there are only a few medicine people left, it was very important to guard your thoughts, especially anything related to sex. Lustful thoughts about another person could really get you into trouble.

Here is story about a young girl whose thinking got her into trouble. I witnessed this event myself when I was a young man of sixteen.

It was 1937 and a group of Dene was camped beside an inland fish lake. One day it was announced that a young girl was very sick. By evening, the family was extremely concerned and asked her brother, a medicine man, to perform a ceremony to discover the source of her illness.

I was very curious about the ceremony. And, as luck would have it for me, their tent was next to ours. My mom and dad planned to go to the ceremony. I announced, "I will be coming, too." Then my mother turned to me and said, "No. You don't know anything about these things so don't go there."

In a short while, I could hear a person singing in the next tent. I was so excited! Although I usually obeyed my parents, this time I could not resist; I wanted to hear and see everything. Silently, I let myself in the tent and sat at the back hoping to go unnoticed. The tent was full of people there to see the ceremony, just like me. It was a fascinating event to watch, even though I could not understand much of what was happening!

The medicine man was singing and mumbling in a strange language that I had never heard before. Now I know that the man was actually in a trance and communicating with the spirit of his medicine power, in the language of that spirit. Each medicine power spirit speaks its own language. During a ceremony like this, the medicine person is in the medicine power world on one level, and can see an image of the medicine-power spirit. At the time, it just seemed very eerie.

Right there, I developed a fascination with medicine power that has driven me all my life. It's why I'm writing this book.

After what seemed like a long time, the man opened his eyes and faced the crowd of people in the tent: "I have learned much today. And I know what has caused my sister's illness. I have been told that I will only be allowed to make medicine power for my sister once in her whole life. If she ever gets sick again, I will not be able to help her. So I must find a way to help her that will last her whole life. I will explain to you what I have learned. Then you, too, can be helped and make sure this never happens to anyone in your family.

"It is normal to think about sex sometimes. It is natural, you could say. But when someone thinks about sex too much or in a way that is not

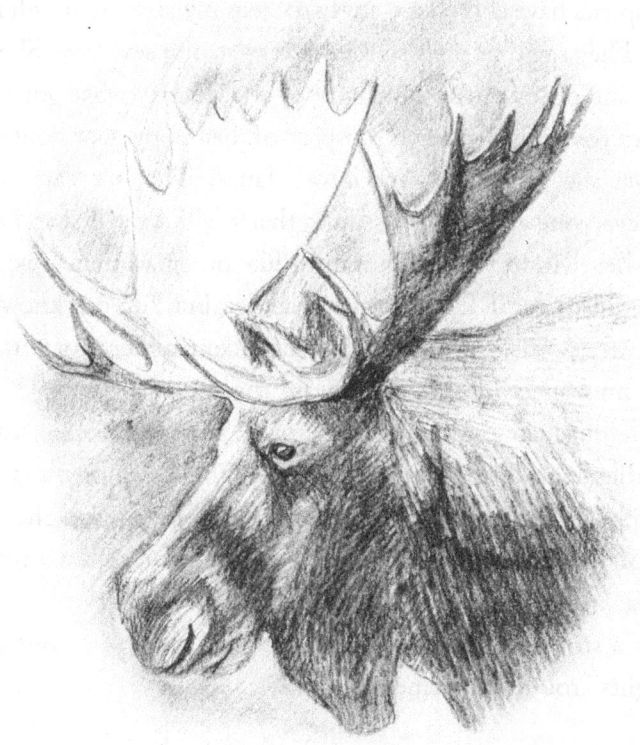

natural, then harm can come to that person. This is what has happened to my sister and it has made her ill. Let me explain.

"One day we brought in some caribou and moose that we had just shot. My sister was given the job to clean the meat and make it ready to cook. As she worked on the dead animal, eventually she had to clean the sex parts of the moose. This started her thinking about the moose and caribou in a sexual way, which is not a natural thing when you are a human being. This went over and over in her mind in all kinds of crazy ways. It became like a sickness with her.

"After some time, the medicine spirit of both the Caribou and the Moose became aware of her obsessive thoughts and were offended by them. They have sent this sickness to her and she will die if I do not intervene.

"The spirits have shown me a way to help my sister that will last her whole life. They say that my sister has a very strong sex drive. She is very young and she obsesses too much about sex. This is what got her into trouble here today. If I change the part of her body that contains her sexual power she will come back into balance. Then she can enjoy life again, like everyone else. But, this thing that I will do will stop her from going into her 'Moon time' each month like other women. I would not want to do this to her if I had any other choice, but I do not know of any other way. Afterwards, she must be taught to control her thoughts and to only entertain respectful thoughts toward the animals."

After he finished speaking to the crowd, he turned to his sister and began another song in the strange language. This ceremony was shorter than the first. When he was done, people left the tent and there was a great deal of talk about this teaching. They say the man's sister recovered fully but was never able to have children.

This is a story of what can happen to you when you don't control your thoughts around medicine power.

20: Medicine Power for Eagle

In the spring of 1926, Paul Blondin was eighty-five years old. Still, he was out hunting beaver and muskrat with his son, Edward. They travelled on a river that flowed into a big lake that had been created through flooding. They maneuvered their canoe through an area where many willows were growing. Late in the morning, Paul said, "Son, I think we should stop and make camp. This rain is miserable weather." They found a spot under the shelter of a big tree and set up camp. They made a fire, skinned some beaver, and went to sleep.

Much later, Edward awoke to find the delicious smell of food cooking and his father sitting beside a crackling fire. Paul said, "Come and eat, my son. The tea is hot. I have something to tell you."

The son got up and sat by his father. His father said, "I didn't sleep at all. An Eagle has a nest in this tree we camped under and as soon as I lay down to sleep he called me. He has brought me some disturbing news. There is a terrible thing happening, a medicine-power war. He says that many medicine people may die, including me, even though it has nothing to do with me. I am sorry to have to tell you this. Let's head back home today. Maybe if I talk to some people it will do some good."

They packed up camp and headed home to the shore of Great Bear Lake where their relatives were camped. Then they prepared to travel by dog team while the ice was still good. They were heading to Fort Franklin one hundred miles away. One week later, they arrived at Fort Franklin. Everything appeared to be well. People were happy playing hand games and holding drum dances.

Paul went straight to the Elders and leaders to have a serious talk. This is what he told them: "I have some very bad news. A serious sickness is coming. It will spread amongst our people and many will die if we don't do something to prevent it. I suggest that we gather our medicine people together. Perhaps if we work together we can stop this terrible

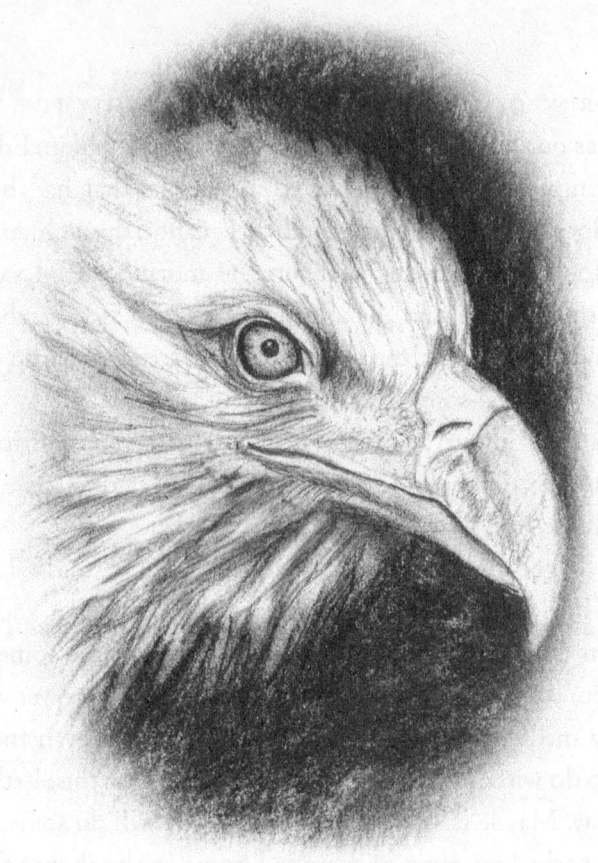

disaster. We should instruct the people to buy what they need at the trading post and then head off into the bush in small groups. They will be safe there when the sickness comes."

The Elders listened quietly to Paul. When he was finished they talked amongst themselves and told him, "Sorry, Paul, but as you can see everything is fine here. People are very happy. We do not see any disaster coming."

Soon even more people arrived at Fort Norman. The dancing and hand games continued until two very powerful medicine people died suddenly. Then many people packed up and headed home to Fort Franklin, but soon the sickness had spread there too. Almost all the Elders and medicine people perished in the influenza epidemic. Sadly, Paul and his older sister died. The flu epidemic of 1926 spread all over the Northwest Territories and was the result of a medicine power conflict between two strong medicine men. The Eagle Spirit's prophecy was fulfilled.

In the past, Dene people experienced disasters but were always able to heal themselves again through medicine power. Then life would continue as before. Since the 1926 epidemic, we have never recovered because the medicine power that was so important to our lifestyle was lost as well. This was the beginning of drastic changes in Dene lifestyle.

21: The Prophecies of Ehtseo Ayah

Our Dene prophet, Ehtseo Ayha, died not long ago, in 1990, at the age of ninety-four. Many people believe in his teachings. Even the Bishop of the area acknowledged that Ayha was a holy man and visited him whenever he travelled nearby.

Ayha taught the people about many things that were yet to come. He said medicine power would disappear not long after he died because the people would no longer take care of it properly. He warned, "You'll just have to do the best you can in the future without medicine power. It does not mean that the Creator has abandoned you. If you continue to pray to the Creator, you will be looked after." He also said, "Very soon you will be forced to change your lifestyle by another people's government. The people will be confused and they will no longer live as we did in the past. You will stop listening to each other. Then your religion will become weak. Still, if you pray to the Creator, your suffering will be eased. Do this for yourself and your people.

I once heard him speak. While pointing to Great Bear Lake, he said, "Soon people will come here and find a rich rock that has never been seen here before. Many people will benefit from this."

We did not know it at the time, but he was predicting the discovery of diamonds in the area.

Ayah was a famous prophet and people travelled a long way to come and listen to him teach. He also received many sacred songs that he sang with his drum. People would come and listen to him talk and sing. They would also pray to the Creator themselves and ask for good health or a long life. Sometimes Ayha would pray for a long time, so the people would also pray for a long time.

22: The Story of Teleway

Teleway was a man from the Colville Lake and Fort Good Hope areas. He was a powerful medicine man, a *Beh Bah Teh*, but he didn't act like other *Beh Bah Teh*. The people considered him to be a great figure. Teleway was well respected wherever he went. He was a great teacher who spent time at gatherings teaching how medicine power works. Teleway was not afraid to talk about medicine power publicly, which is how this information reached even the poorest people who did not possess medicine powers. Teleway understood medicine power because he was a medicine man. Unlike others, he was willing to share his knowledge openly. This made him a great person in people's eyes.

He had knowledge of sacred medicine power. He taught that there is a Creator and that all people should pray to Him. The Creator is for everybody. The Creator is the most powerful spirit in the universe and knows everyone. If you talk or think to the Creator, He will know. He advised us to talk—or think—to the Creator and ask for what we want: a favour, good luck, long life, and so on. If you truly believe in the Creator, He will know you are there and listen to you. Teleway spoke a great deal about the Creator.

The first missionaries who came into the area found our people receptive to the teachings of the church and were able to convert them readily because we already believed in the Creator. Teleway taught that medicine power is a gift from the Creator. It is created for us to use in our life to survive. Medicine power ownership has to be managed in the right way. It does not come to a person with the intention that they do anything they like with it. It is not that way.

Medicine power has laws that must be followed by all people all the time. In order to do things the right way with medicine power, which is still the property of the Creator, it can be very difficult. Teleway talked about everything regarding medicine power. Whenever there were children at a gathering, he would teach them about medicine power. Teleway was a good man. His life is legendary, and many people still talk about him.

When the world was new, in the beginning of Creation, medicine power was created along with the animals and human beings. Medicine power is a spirit. The great medicine-power people are all involved with spirits. Each medicine person owns or possesses a specific kind—or kinds—of medicine power that he or she uses to make medicine.

A medicine person communicates with the spirits. They can see, hear, and talk to spirits, including the spirits of people who have passed away. Sometimes when a person dies, one of their relatives may want to know what happened to their loved one's spirit. They may approach a medicine person who has the ability to follow a spirit's path, and the medicine person can tell the relatives what happened to the deceased person's spirit. They may even tell them that their loved one has reincarnated into another life.

Teleway was such a person. Teleway was reincarnated three times and could remember each successive incarnation. He told stories about his previous lives and claimed that he could remember everything. His medicine power remained with him in each life.

In his first life, he was born just before the fur traders arrived in the area. He was still alive when the fur traders established a trading post along the Mackenzie River near what we now call Fort Good Hope. This was the area where Teleway lived. He had a long life. He had strong medicine power for spirits and did a lot of work for people tracing people's spirit paths. Finally, when he was very old, lying in his deathbed, he told his family, "Don't cry for me. I will live a second time on Mother Earth. So don't feel bad for me when I die." After he died, the people remembered what he said and asked a strong medicine power man to investigate what happened to Teleway's spirit.

The medicine man traced Teleway's spirit to a pregnant woman. He told the people, "If that woman has a baby boy, that will be Teleway reincarnating into a second life." The woman delivered a boy who they called Teleway Number Two. He was born the second time when the fur buyers were pretty strong in the country. Fort Good Hope had two trading posts and Colville Lake had even more. It is one hundred and ten miles from Colville Lake to Fort Good Hope.

Dene people were poor in those days. In November, after the first furs were trapped, they would begin the long journey to Fort Good Hope to trade for things they needed. When Teleway was nineteen years old, he and another man his age decided to walk to Fort Good Hope. They expected the trip to take three days. The boys packed carefully for the long journey, said goodbye to their relatives, and started off. However, that was the last the families ever saw of the boys. They never returned. A search party was established to look for the boys, but they were never found. People believed the boys likely fell through thin ice and drowned.

Three years later, around Easter, the weather was warm and many people were in town. Soon a large gathering began to take shape. The people came together while Elders took turns talking to the people. In the crowd sat a woman with a three-year-old baby. He turned to his mother and began to talk. He pointed his small fingers at one old man sitting in the crowd. He told his mother, "He shot me," and pointed his finger at the old man.

The mother grabbed the baby and took him home. There she fed him. When he was settled down, she took him to a quiet place and asked him, "Why did you say that the old man shot you?" Then the baby said, "My name is Teleway. I remember my friend and me walking on the ice when we met an old man. As we approached his cabin, he pulled out a rifle and shot us both. I left my body with the spirit of my medicine power. Then I observed what the old man did to our bodies. He put our bodies in an old canvas bag with many rocks inside. Then he cut a hole in the ice and let our bodies sink there. I was so mad, I found a pregnant woman right away. I got into her womb and I was born right away. I truly am Teleway. This happened three years ago."

The mother of that baby was really disturbed by what she heard, so she told her mother and dad what her son had said. They gathered a group of Elders that were related to the late Teleway, his original mother and father, and other important Elders and group leaders. They gathered in the baby's tent. They treated the baby very well. Once again he told what happened to him. The group was surprised that a small baby of three years old could talk so well. The Elders said that he must be a strong medicine-power person to be able to tell someone what happened to him three years ago in another life.

So the group agreed to do something about it: "Let's not rush. We will do it the right way and confront the old man. Then we can see how he reacts. First, let's find two good medicine-power people that deal with spirits and ghosts to find out if this baby is really Teleway."

Later that day, they had two medicine-power people trace the baby's spirit. They confirmed that the baby was, in fact, Teleway, who reincarnated on earth a third time. The group decided that the next day they would all go out and gather together as many people as possible.

Teleway's relatives went out and invited many people to the meeting. They were happy to come because Teleway was widely respected. With a large gathering established, the old man was invited to attend. He still hadn't heard the reason for the gathering. Seating was arranged so that the mother and the baby were sitting in the middle of the tent among the other women; the Elders sat in the front row, and they placed the old man nearby. A speaker addressed the crowd that was gathered: "We have an unusual reason for meeting today. I ask that you listen carefully to all that is said here today. Three years ago, a young man named Teleway and his friend disappeared while on a journey from Colville Lake to this place. We never saw them again. Now we think we have information about what happened to Teleway. This is what we want to speak about here today. Can you face this woman here with her child beside her? They have something to tell you. Please listen carefully."

With the entire group facing and listening to the pair, the mother began to question her son. "My baby, what is your name?"

He answered in a voice that seemed older than his few years: "My name is Teleway."

She asked him, "Tell me what happened to you."

He said, "I got shot."

She asked, "Who did it?"

Then Teleway pointed his tiny finger at the old man: "That man shot me and my friend a long time ago. We were walking on the lake. Just as we approached the shore, he shot us. We just wanted to camp with him. He shot us for no reason. As soon as I got hit, my spirit left my body. Then I watched what the old man was doing to our bodies. He cut a hole in the ice. Then he put our bodies and many rocks in a canvas bag. Then he put us down that hole."

The child continued, "I was so mad I wanted to be born again. I found a pregnant woman—my mother. I was born right away. It's been three years since I was killed. I am three years old."

There was an uproar in the tent. Everyone seemed to be talking all at once. Some were yelling. Someone grabbed the old man and shouted, "Let's kill him!" One of the Elders raised his voice and said, "Everyone quiet down. Let's do things slowly."

Finally the group calmed down. One person confronted the old man and asked him, "Is it true that you killed the boys?"

The old man admitted it. He said, "I don't know what came over me. I just loaded my gun and shot at them. I didn't even know who they were at the time."

One of the Elders, a relative of Teleway's said, "We are related to the boys. We will go with the old man to his camp and he can show us where he put them. Then we can take the bones and give them a proper burial. We will leave the old man alone. Killing him will not change what happened. Besides, he is an old man. He will only live a few years."

Later in life, Teleway Number Three was recognized as a strong and good medicine-power person. He was a quiet man who was always willing to help another. Still, his reputation as a strong medicine-power person attracted many, many people to him, and this was hard for him at times. People truly never left him alone.

This is one of the sacrifices that is required of medicine-power people, which can become a heavy burden. Edwar, of the Delta, once fled his area because he was so overwhelmed with the number of people who asked for his help.

It was the same for Teleway. This also explains why medicine power people are usually quiet and rarely talk publicly about their own medicine power. They are different from others because medicine power is a spirit, and to own medicine power you have to be careful. That is why they are that way.

When the world was new, two out of every ten people possessed medicine power. All people believed in medicine power because they could see it in action in their everyday lives. Besides, their whole lives depended on medicine power. When someone had a problem, a dispute with someone else, or a sickness in their family, they would turn to a person with medicine power for help. That is why medicine-power people were very busy with requests from others. Even if someone had never seen medicine power work before, they still had to trust medicine people because sometimes that was all there was to solve their problems.

Some people think medicine can do everything, but this is not the case. A medicine power person can only help with the medicine power that he or she possesses. There are some problems people have that can't be helped unless a medicine power person who possesses that specific kind of power can be found.

Medicine power is limited. An individual only receives the kind of medicine power that the Creator gives him or her. Teleway healed many sick people but only when he had the kind of medicine power needed for that particular sickness. If he had no power for it he couldn't help.

With regards to the health of a human body, there are many, many different kinds of illnesses that could kill a person. In some ways, a modern doctor and a medicine power person are the same. For both of them, when they fail to heal a sick person it is because it is beyond them to help.

For example, if a boy has an illness that has the potential to be fatal, a doctor who identifies the illness may be able to cut it out or give the right kind of medicine to help the patient. This is true with medicine power as well. If a medicine-power person possesses three hundred different kinds of medicine power that heal the body, he most likely would be able to help the patient. But if he has only ten kinds of medicine power for healing, he only works with the ten different kinds. If the illness requires a different kind of medicine power, the patient will not be healed.

Generally, medicine power is limited. Teleway helped many sick people whenever he could. He was very good at healing infected wounds by making medicine for the person. Another ability that he was good at was tracing the path of a spirit. He would trace a spirit and report back to the individual who requested the information. He also had wind medicine power.

23: Medicine Power for the Wind

Teleway and many of his people died long ago. In 1926, a terrible flu epidemic spread throughout the area. It was then that Aboriginal people lost most of their medicine people. Teleway and Paul Blondin, from Fort Norman, NWT, were good friends. They both passed away during that epidemic.

The Hudson Bay Company used to hire strong people to make the long trip from the north down the waterways toward Edmonton. They used York boats. There was one boat was for each community on the Mackenzie River. There were many Dene who were working on the York boats. It is a very long journey from the Delta to the southern waterways, which is approximately two thousand miles of river.

Both Teleway and Paul Blondin were working on the same York boat. In fact, many medicine-power people worked together on that trip. As they paddled up the strong river, they got so tired that they asked the medicine men to make the wind blow behind them. Some people are able to do that, but usually the wind blows for only a short time.

First they paddled up the river. Then, when they came out onto the Great Slave Lake, they noticed that there was no wind at all. The water was very calm. Everyone was very tired and hungry, so they landed on an island to make lunch. Sometimes, when someone paddles as hard and long as they had, they get very bad blisters. If the blisters break, they can bleed. It's very painful. The willow tree is helpful for treating this kind of injury. A willow must be cut, then heated over the fire, and finally rubbed on the blister. This will harden the skin.

So after they ate lunch, this is what they proceeded to do. Some of the group lay down to have a little rest. But Teleway noticed his younger brother's hands were bleeding, so he prepared a willow to help him. Then he lay down as well.

Usually, when a medicine power person intends to make the wind blow, he will sing or yell. But Teleway spoke in a quiet voice and said, "Why does a small thing like that have to make my brother suffer like this?"

Then, suddenly, the wind started to blow behind them. People jumped up and rushed to load their boats. They yelled out, "Put up the sail!" Still, the wind blew harder and the boat went faster. The group was afraid to stop and make fire for fear that the wind would stop. The Great Slave Lake is one hundred miles across. The trip up the Slave River to the rapids at Fort Smith, NWT, is another one hundred and fifty miles.

The group had a good rest. It was the first time they could actually sleep in the boat. In no time, they made it across the lake but still the wind blew so they continued up the Slave River. The river is very crooked up there, but still the wind blew even harder so they travelled very fast. They travelled two hundred and fifty miles from the island the day before. They landed at Fort Smith without a problem.

That whole summer the experience continued. When Teleway would get to shore to eat or sleep, the wind would stop. Then, as soon as he got back into the boat, the wind would start to blow behind them. They would put up the sail and continue on their travels. This pattern continued until Teleway got home to Fort Good Hope in October when the snow began to fall. He was the greatest man to be able to make the wind blow behind them like that all summer long. People all over the Mackenzie Valley talked about it for a long time.

How can a medicine man make the wind blow? First, as I have already explained, they have to possess medicine power for wind, such as Teleway did. He had a complete knowledge of wind medicine power from the very beginning. He understood how the wind was created and understood the power of wind. He knew exactly how the wind worked. He had all the necessary medicine power to take action with the wind.

Teleway was a good man, a gentle person, who never caused a problem to others. He spent his whole life with the people from the Fort Good Hope area, and they have never forgotten him. They still tell many stories about him and how he helped people during his ninety years of life.

What I find the most unusual about him is that he lived three times on Mother Earth and could remember each of his lives and wasn't afraid to talk about it. He's an exceptional person to remember and talk about.

24: Monster Medicine Power

TODAY, THE LIFESTYLE OF DENE PEOPLE IS VERY DIFFERENT THAN in times past. One of the changes is that medicine power is being extinguished. When the world was new, Dene people based their lifestyle on medicine power. When something happened that they didn't understand, they would use medicine power to uncover the answer.

At times, a parent may recognize something in their baby or small child that seemed unusual. Then they would seek out a medicine-power person to determine whether or not the baby possessed medicine power. If the child was found to possess medicine power, the medicine person would counsel the parents to be very careful with how they raised their baby. Some medicine people would not only be able to determine if the baby had medicine power, but also what kind of power. This is very deep work.

In Colville Lake, in the 1900s, a mother once asked a medicine person to determine whether her son had medicine power. She felt he didn't act like a normal baby. The medicine man agreed and carried out the ceremony. Her suspicions were confirmed. Then one of her relatives asked the medicine person to find out what kind of medicine power the baby owned. So the next day the medicine person performed another ceremony.

He reported that the baby owned a type of monster medicine power. This monster was the strongest animal on earth, and to have medicine power for such a thing could be dangerous. Many people were present at the ceremony including a number of Elders. The medicine man told the parents, "Take extra care of this baby because he is very special."

Over the years, they had other children, until they had four boys and one girl. The medicine man performed the ceremony on all four boys and discovered that they all had monster medicine power.

Aboriginal people who lived during those times understood medicine power. They acknowledged that medicine power is a gift from the Creator, and everyone needed it to survive. Our lives depended on it. All Aboriginal people were to strictly follow medicine-power law, and with it we lived very well. It was everyone's responsibility to use medicine power wisely because, when used in the wrong way, it could be very dangerous.

The medicine man who performed the ceremony on the four boys was considered very credible and reliable. Still, it was rare for four children from one family to have the same type of medicine power, particularly monster medicine power. The whole village of Colville Lake was in an uproar, worrying and talking about the news. The Elders gathered to discuss it again and again.

The medicine people explained to the village, "Monster medicine power is not new. Other people have had monster medicine, too. A monster is the strongest animal on Earth. If a man has monster medicine power, he could be a very dangerous person if he uses it to harm others."

The Elders told people who came to listen to the discussions about the boys, "These children should be treated very carefully by everyone in the community as they grow from children to adults. If one of the brothers treats others the wrong way, they could cause a grave conflict with medicine power, or create many enemies, or even a war. It is important for the future of our people that these brothers are treated well. Treat the boys with care. Try not to make them mad. Be careful not to hurt their feelings and be very polite to them."

The village Elders were concerned about what might happen some day if the boys were not raised in the right way. The Elders then counseled the boys' parents about how to raise them. They said, "It is important to raise them very carefully right from the time they start to talk. It would be best for you to live alone in the bush, away from others. Keep them away from other children. The most important thing to remember is to keep them happy. Laugh as much as you can and try to avoid things that make them angry."

So, in an act of great sacrifice, the family moved into isolation where they lived for the next twenty years. In later years, their mother recalled, "I made up my mind to raise my boys according to what the Elders told me. I was so busy looking after them that I didn't even have time to do women's chores. I had to concentrate on the boys steadily. I always needed at least one other woman staying there to help me. There was my grandmother, my older sister, my younger sister, and many other women throughout those twenty years.

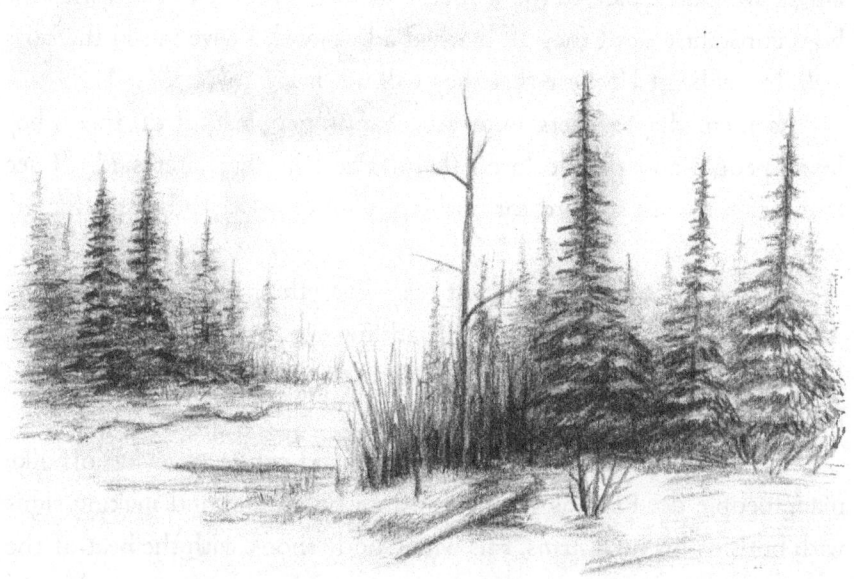

"I remember once when the oldest one was about eight years old. It was a hot summer day. I sat down on the lakeshore with them to watch and make sure they didn't fight or get mad. There we were, sitting on the bank. Next thing you know, they were yelling away. One of the boys, who was only three years old at the time and could barely walk, picked up a big ball of stone almost bigger than him. I looked up to see what they were yelling about and I saw him holding that stone. It must have been fifty pounds. A grown man couldn't have lifted that stone, yet the baby was holding it up in the air like a toy. He threw the boulder in the water and they were all yelling because water splashed on them. They thought it was funny. But it wasn't for me. I grabbed my baby and played with him until he started to laugh.

"I saw my four boys do a lot of things that nobody else could do. I used to worry so much about them. I was afraid that they might kill somebody someday. The hardest time was when they were teenagers. I had to prevent them from talking to each other harshly and fighting. I did all kinds of things to make them happy. I was always making them laugh, telling jokes. I danced with them. I invented games to make them laugh. We played ball. In the winter, I sledded with them. I was with the boys constantly until they all reached adulthood. I have raised the boys well. In my heart I believe that they will not harm anyone."

As men, the brothers were very happy people, full of fun. They loved people and people loved them. Their mother later said, "I see that I didn't work so hard for nothing. I am glad that I did this for my boys."

The brothers were great, giant men. Everything about them was big. They were tall, had big heads, big sparkling eyes, and wide, strong arms. In 1921, my mom and dad saw one of them at a large gathering on the Barren lands.

She said, "This brother was playing hand games, showing off like many people do. He was yelling and moving around and making signs with both of his huge arms. His whole body shook with the beat of the drum. He was a good player and wonderful to watch. People came from all over just to see this giant of a man play."

Their mother was so happy to see her boys have a lot of fun. They came to be good boys.

25: Monster Medicine Power II

THE BOYS LIVED LONG LIVES, AND, FOR THE MOST PART, THEIR LIVES were without incident. However, two unfortunate events occurred throughout their lives. The first incident resulted in tragedy.

In time, all of the four boys got married. One morning, one of the brothers got up and went to visit Adam, a small-time medicine man from Fort Good Hope, who, as it turned out, was visiting his nets right at that time. When the brother saw that Adam was not there, he returned to his own tent and wife and lay down for a nap. A short while later Adam burst through the door full of accusations. He said, "You think you are the only one with monster medicine power. Well, you're not! I have the same kind of power. You were bothering my wife today when I was away and I don't like it. Let's fight it out!"

Then Adam jumped on him and grabbed him by the throat. The brother became very angry when he heard Adam's accusation and threat. In a second, he transformed into monster medicine power in spirit. He grabbed Adam by the chest and got up. It seemed there was no time to even go through the doorway, so he just went right through the tent wall. The tent was in shreds as they continued to fight outside.

The brother swung Adam in the air like he was just a rag. You could hear the crack of Adam's bones breaking. People were screaming, "He's going to kill Adam!"

A quick-thinking Elder told a boy, "Go get his brothers! They're the only ones who can stop him now!"

His brothers eventually stopped the fight. But it was too late for Adam: his back was broken, his hip was dislocated, and one leg was broken, as was one arm. The fight was over, but Adam's injuries were life threatening. A group of Elders spoke to the four brothers. They said, "Only one thing can save Adam now." Later that night the brothers made medicine power over Adam and saved his life.

However, poor Adam was greatly disfigured. He had a crooked back, and a terrible limp from the injury to his hip. One leg was shorter than the other. His whole body shook badly for the rest of his life. Adam really suffered. Still, it was his own fault, for if he hadn't started the fight, none of this would have happened to him.

The second incident happened when one of the brothers was out hunting caribou at the edge of the Barren lands. He shot a big bull caribou, butchered it, and packed it up to carry back to camp. The wind was strong and the pack was heavy, even for such a powerful man. He struggled with his load and his footing in the dim light of the evening sky. Then a grave misfortune happened: the brother actually stepped on a grizzly bear that had been asleep in the willows.

Both animal and man were very surprised. The alarmed bear jumped up and charged the man. When a bear is mad, his claws come foreward, long and sharp. He dug into the man's head and pulled his scalp completely off. The brother fell to the ground with his pack still on his back. But there was no time to lose. He was fighting for his life. In a heartbeat, he transformed into a monster spirit. When you are a spirit, things can happen extremely fast.

The rope that tied the pack together—including the head strap—was made of braided moose hide. It is used because it is so strong that it cannot be broken. When the man fell down, the rope fell around his neck. The weight of the meat pulled him down on top of the grizzly bear. By that time, the bear was fighting mad.

With enormous force, and the use of monster medicine power, the man broke the rope as if it were a piece of twine. Then, with one arm, he grabbed the bear's chest and pushed himself up with the other arm. He grasped the bear's nose and twisted his head—until he broke the bear's neck and tore the bear's head from his body. Then, in an act of triumph, he actually threw the head away.

How could the bear be alive when he had no head? That is how the man killed the bear to save himself. He crawled around until he found his scalp, tied it to his head, which was bleeding profusely, and attempted to walk back to camp and his waiting wife. When he finally couldn't make it any farther, he shot his gun to alert his wife.

By then it was dark. His wife heard the shooting and went out to look for him. Eventually she found him in a pitiful state. She helped him back to camp. The next day, she found the other brothers who were camped not too far away. They gathered in one camp and stayed together until the brother was well again. He lived a long life.

The only disfigurement he suffered was a big, black scar right above his eyes where they sewed his scalp back on his head. This made him look especially dangerous, mean, and ugly. People were afraid just to see him. Then the story of how he killed a grizzly bear with his bare hands spread, and he became a legend that we still talk about today.

Many people were scared of the brothers because they were well known for their monster medicine power. But, in truth, they were good men: polite, well-mannered, full of fun and jokes, and made people laugh.

26: Comparing Medicine Power

IT'S IMPORTANT TO UNDERSTAND THAT EVEN THOUGH TWO MEDICINE-power people may own the same kind of medicine power, they may not have equal power. It depends on how they received medicine power in the first place. For example, let's say a moose has three hundred different body parts. If a person has medicine power for those three hundred parts of the moose, he would be a 100 per cent master medicine power person for moose. He could make a moose do anything he wants. But it's very seldom you find a master medicine power.

You are more likely to find a medicine-power person with a small number of items of moose medicine power. Still, if he has medicine power for the moose's brain, he could control the moose's mind. Even though that is only one item, he would still be the best moose hunter in the country.

Three different medicine power people could have a different number of items of medicine power, even though they may all possess medicine power for moose. One could have five items, one could have thirty items, and one could have forty items. They may all seem the same, if you only considered that they all possess medicine power for moose; however, they are not equal. Still, they all have moose medicine power and could do a great deal to help other people. This is true of all kinds of medicine power, such as animals, plants, insects, rocks—all things on earth and in space and everything else.

In the case of the brothers with medicine power for monsters, it is told that all four boys had 100 per cent power for monster medicine. It is highly unusual for four people in one family to have 100 per cent of any kind of medicine power, especially monster medicine. But that is what people claimed they had.

A medicine person could own any number of virtually billions of different items of medicine power. Some get only a few items, and others seem to receive too much. Dene people believe that there is one Creator who created everything on earth and in space—even this complicated topic: medicine power. There are billions of different items of medicine power and millions of people who may receive the medicine power.

Yamoria and Edwar were two medicine people who possessed a very high level of medicine. It was what is called "sacred medicine power." Yamoria and Edwar possessed sacred knowledge about the Creator and shared this with the people through their teachings. The four brothers who had monster medicine power also had knowledge of sacred medicine power, even though they did not possess it themselves. Over many years, they received daily visits from spirit helpers in visions that taught them these sacred things.

In time, the brothers got old but had also learned a great deal about sacred medicine power, which they spoke about to the people at gatherings. They taught about the Creator and medicine power. It seemed that they were not afraid to talk about medicine power, which was unusual. They explained, in simple terms, how medicine power works and assured the people that the Creator gave us medicine power to help each other.

They explained that visions from spirit helpers teach a medicine-power person from the time he or she is a small child. It begins at an early age to help that person understand and deal with the experiences that they are having. For example, it is common for a medicine person to see all kinds of spirits. Some of them look dangerous, which could easily frighten a child if he or she did not understand what was happening. Also, this education is important to teach children how to manage the medicine power they possess. They say, after a time, it becomes easy to discuss anything with the medicine-power spirit.

The brothers explained, "Many people come to us asking for our help and we help when we can. We are different from other medicine-power people who possess medicine power that makes them the best hunter, trapper, or fisherman. They use their medicine power to help feed the people. But that is quite different than when people come to us for healing.

"When you need healing, you have to ask a medicine person who possesses an item of medicine power for the human body, or an animal, an insect, or some combination that is required for the sickness that you need healed. However, we only have one item of medicine power: monster medicine power. Still we have medicine power for every item of the monster body, so, for example, if a person has a liver illness, we could use monster liver medicine power. This may heal the person. When we help people heal, we use medicine power from the monster body part. It doesn't always help. When we are trying to heal a person, we are actually asking for help from the medicine power. Many people think we are causing the healing, but, in fact, it is the medicine power.

"Our spirit helpers have explained many things to us. We know the Creator exists and that there are laws that we should follow on this earth. Those rare people who received sacred medicine power see the spirit of this power at all times. The spirit counsels them about how to teach the people. Some receive sacred songs to sing with their drum. Then they teach the people these special songs for them to use."

Many groups still sing these sacred songs today. Even the people who hear the songs seem to be able to pray better to the Creator. Praying in this way has always been an important element of Dene culture.

When the missionaries arrived in the north, they did not approve of the Dene people's religious practices. They tried to stop them praying with the drum and song by claiming that it was evil. But it was so strong that the Dene refused to give it up.

As the brothers got old, they preached a great deal about the Creator. Even though they never did receive sacred medicine power, they still had reliable information from their many visions. They became devout followers of the teachings of sacred medicine power, in their old age. They spent all their time at gatherings where they could teach the people about these things.

The Dene people learned a great deal about how medicine power works from people like the brothers, who were so eager to share this knowledge. They taught us that medicine power is a gift from the Creator who intended us to use it to help each other. They also taught that there are medicine-power laws that must be followed.

In the time that the brothers lived, many people feared they would harm others with their medicine power. Instead, they helped many people and contributed to the knowledge of the people. There are many lessons within the story of the four brothers who possessed monster medicine power.

27: A Powerful Medicine Person as Leader

In times past, Dene people loved and depended on medicine power for their survival. They also feared it. That is one reason why the people often made a strong medicine person their leader. It made them feel safer. They depended on their leader to protect them from other medicine people who would use bad medicine. If a strong medicine-power person lived in the village, the people were safe. They knew that other nations would not consider attacking them when a powerful medicine person was ready to defend the people.

It's been told that one strong medicine-power person was capable of killing several hundred people. Everyone recognized that it was dangerous to attack a village if there was a strong medicine-power person living there.

When a strong medicine person was a leader and honestly and sincerely wanted to help the people, he or she could provide great assistance to others. He or she could urge people to follow Dene law, heal the sick, hunt or fish, resolve conflicts between married couples, and even investigate crimes such as murder. Therefore, it was very important to have a strong medicine person as your leader.

28: War Using Medicine Power

WHEN THE WORLD WAS NEW AND THE CHIPEWYAN NATION HAD established contact with the European fur traders, they acquired items such as steel knives and axes, matches and cloth. Still, some northern tribes, like the Rabbitskin Nation, had never seen a "white man." They continued to live as they had for many generations, finding all that they needed to survive from the land. It was a time when medicine power was strong and abundant. People travelled all over to harvest what they needed from the land. They relied on medicine power to survive and help each other.

The Chipewyan Nation occupied the area around Lake Athabasca, north to the Barren lands and west through northern Saskatchewan. They followed the caribou herd in a way similar to the Inuit. Sometimes they were even seen on the north side of the Great Bear Lake, which is fifteen hundred miles away. They had strong medicine-power people and warriors, and they worked hard together.

The Rabbitskin Nation, from what is now called Colville Lake, was also a large group that travelled throughout the area. They hunted on the Barren lands for caribou, which they used for food and clothing. Like other tribes, caribou was necessary for their survival.

During the time of this story, the Rabbitskin Nation sent hunters to the Barren lands for caribou. However, they found that a number of their hunters failed to return to the larger group. Parties were sent out to search for them, but they couldn't be found. Scouts did find signs of other people hunting in the area, but they were not Rabbitskin people. This worried them.

They discussed what to do. They said, "We have the whole summer to contact each other if we lose anybody from now on. But perhaps it is best for us to travel to our home territory quickly and forget about the caribou hunting for now."

The Rabbitskin people had powerful medicine people who could perform a ceremony that would explain what happened to the hunters. Many people claimed that their medicine people were the most powerful around. They said, "The Chipewyans are responsible for the disappearance of our hunters."

It was decided that it was dangerous for Rabbitskin people to be out on the Barren lands at that time. The group headed back to their home territory. Still, there were about four families who decided to stay behind to take advantage of the good hunting.

One day, a young Rabbitskin man came stumbling up to a family group of twelve hunters who had decided to continue hunting on the Barren lands. He had a terrifying tale to tell of how all his family were slaughtered by a group of Chipewyan warriors. He was the only survivor. The place where they were slain is now called "Bloody River."

This alarmed the group because just that day they had seen a Chipewyan warrior near their camp. They feared that the Chipewyans would try to attack them during the night. Later, as the sun set, they could hear signs of the enemy nearby. They gathered together to devise a plan. They asked within the group if anyone had medicine power that could help. Finally, an Elder said, "I have medicine power for fog if you think that would help."

They were desperate so they told him, "Yes, make some fog!"

He started singing immediately. His words were elaborate and told the story of how fog was created in the beginning. When he finished, a thick fog appeared. He told the people, "Start packing right away. Leave

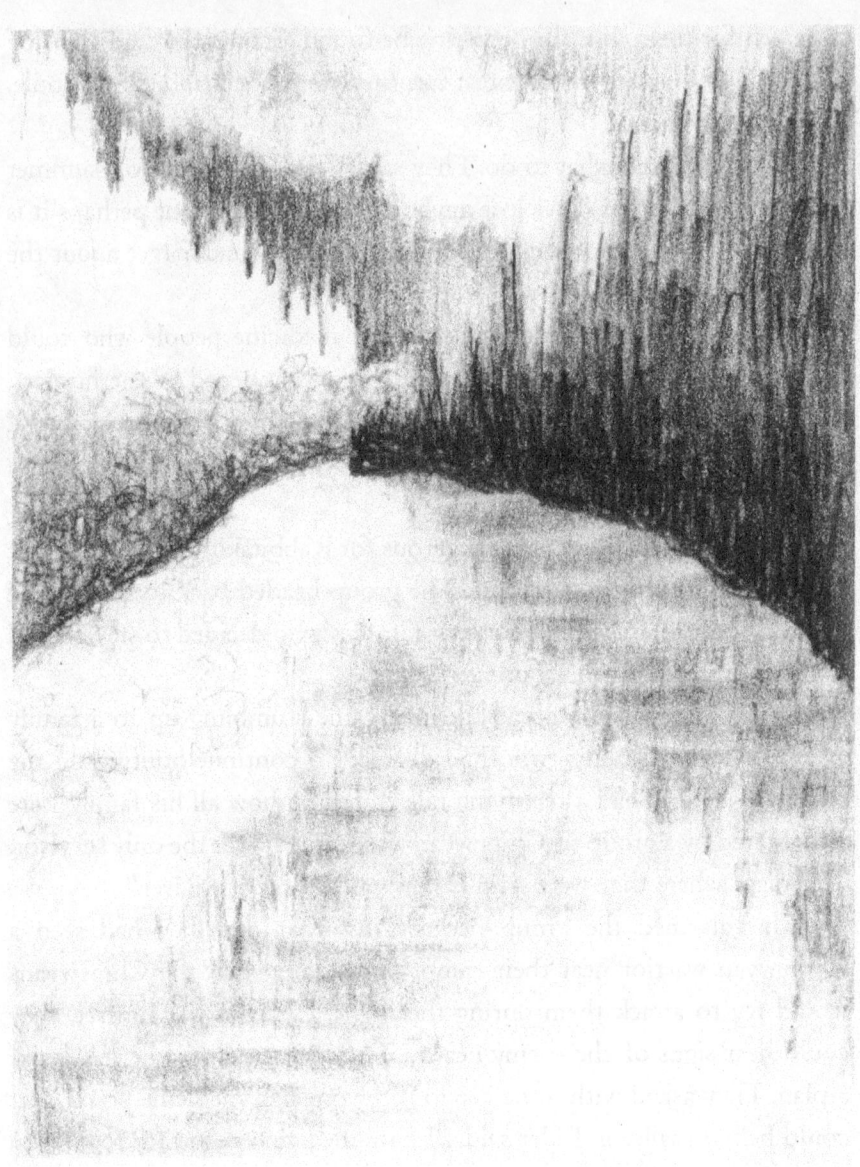

anything heavy. Our lives are at stake. Pack very lightly; we'll be running. Let's tie all the ropes together. Then you can hold on to the rope and I will lead you through the fog to safety. Don't say a word." The fog was so thick they couldn't see where they were walking.

A Chipewyan guard was watching their camp because they intended to attack the Rabbitskin people at daylight. He noticed movement in the thick fog and realized that they must be leaving. He tried to tell the rest of his group, but it was so dark and foggy that he could not find his way. He started to shout out, "They're leaving! They're getting away!"

With that, the Rabbitskin people ran even faster, still holding onto the rope, single file, following the medicine man. It was so dark and foggy that they couldn't see where they were stepping. They couldn't even see their own feet. They just held on and ran for their lives.

They could hear the enemy yelling, but the sound faded after a while. The Chipewyans were so lost in the dark and fog that they had to yell and yell to try to find each other. After a while, the Rabbitskin group heard nothing, but they kept running all night long. By the next day when the sun was high in the sky, the fog finally lifted. Then they were able to recognize landmarks that were familiar. Soon they were in their home territory with the rest of their relatives.

Around the same time, there were two brothers hunting alone. The younger brother was wild and didn't listen well to his older brother. They hoped to kill two or three caribou to make dry meat and tan new hides. But they were having a difficult time finding the herd, so they kept on travelling.

The oldest brother told the younger, "The enemy is around here, so let's be careful where we walk in the Barren lands. If the enemy sees us they are sure to attack."

Unfortunately, the younger brother wouldn't listen.

Just as they reached a hilltop, they looked down into the valley to see a crowd of people walking in line. The younger brother went to yell out to the group, but the oldest brother stopped him: "Quiet! Sit down. They might be the enemy!"

Out of sight, they sat and watched the group make camp. Then they crept up as close as they dared to get a better look. The older brother whispered, "Yes, I'm sure of it. They are the enemy. If they see us they will kill us. We'd better go home and let our people know that we have seen an enemy camp."

Just then, a robin landed on a rock near by and started to squawk. A robin will sound an alert when they observe something approaching. The Chipewyan knew this.

Abruptly, the Chipewyans stood up and started to look for what the robin had seen. Two men grabbed their weapons and began to search the area, walking directly toward the two brothers. The brothers were numb with fear. They were trapped. If they tried to run away they would be seen.

The oldest brother looked down to see his younger brother weeping silently in terror. Filled with heartache and rage, his mind raced for a way to save them. He immediately called upon his medicine power for help. As the two Chipewyan walked closer and closer, he began his ceremony. He quietly spoke the elaborate verse that pleaded with the medicine power spirit of the sun for help.

In an instant, the sun got so bright it was difficult to see. He urged his younger brother, "Put your head down and—no matter what happens—don't open your eyes." The two Chipewyans were almost upon the brothers, but the bright sun was blinding them. They turned away for some relief and headed back to their camp rubbing their eyes.

The brothers returned home safely that summer, although many of the Rabbitskin hunters did not. The Rabbitskin Nation was large at that time. Their territory, the Colville Lake area, is a huge land mass filled with lakes. At that time, the lakes were teeming with fish. There were many ducks, beaver, muskrat, and big game. It was a rich, abundant land.

When the caribou hunters returned with the news that the enemy had killed many of the hunters, there was great anguish and distress among the people. They sent runners to any nearby groups of Rabbitskin people with this message: "Chipewyan warriors have killed many of our hunters out on the Barren lands. Come. We will have a council and decide what to do. We need your best medicine-power people."

They came and they met. Some of the leaders said, "They cannot do whatever they want with us. We are not dead. We are human beings. They will not get away with murdering our people."

They enlisted five of the best medicine-power people they had to find out where the enemy had come from and how strong they were with medicine power. They wanted to find out if they could overpower them with their own medicine.

The medicine-power people made a ceremony. After a long time of singing and quietly reciting the elaborate verses, they gave their report to the people: "These people are a Chipewyan tribe far from their own area. A large group of Chipewyan live all over the main Barren lands. They live like the Inuit. This group lives between the Great Bear Lake and the Coppermine River. They are not too far from where our people hunt, and there are more groups that went further north. A great many of them live in an area of land that stretches all the way to the north end of Saskatchewan. They now occupy lands that are about fifteen hundred miles away from their original area."

The Elders asked, "How strong is their medicine power and do we have medicine to overpower them?"

The five medicine-power people went back to conduct another ceremony. It was a long time before they were finished and ready to report to the people. They announced, "Yes, we can overpower them and make medicine power that will control their minds. We will make them think that the Rabbitskin Nation intends to make peace with them. But we do not. We intend to have revenge. They murdered our people and now they will pay.

"We will make them think that they want peace with us and they will travel to us. So, soon they will arrive. We have a large group of strong medicine-power people. Be ready, and when they arrive we will kill them."

The Rabbitskin people moved to a large fish lake on a common route to Colville Lake. Then they chose strong medicine-power people and warriors and waited. Soon after freeze up, the first group arrived. There were only five of them and the Rabbitskin quickly killed them.

The second group came around December. There were eight of them and the Rabbitskin people killed them easily. The third group came in March when the days are long. Behzie was the leader of the Rabbitskin tribe. He was a powerful man with medicine power. A group of Rabbitskin warriors waited at the fish lake. They were not afraid, for they were sure that they could overpower them with medicine power and control their minds.

The last group of Chipewyans to arrive had a leader by the name of Ah Beh Cho. There were ten of them. This group was different than the rest in that it included some of the Chipewyan's strong medicine-power people. The Chipewyans had contact with the fur traders, which meant that they carried big knives, blankets, an axe, matches, and other things. Some of the items the Rabbitskin people had never even seen before.

When this group of Chipewyans arrived at the fish lake, they had a different attitude than the other groups. They approached the meeting with suspicion and caution. They were very direct and identified why they were there right away.

Ah Beh Cho said, "We are looking for some of our people. We have been wondering why they have not returned from their journey to make peace with you. Can you explain why you have some cloth that belongs to our people? Have you harmed them?"

Behzie answered him cleverly, "We are here to fish for a large crowd that is at the main fish lake. We made peace with others from your nation and then we had a great feast, drum dance, and gift exchange to show our friendship. Some of your people exchanged small things like knives and cloth."

However, the Chipewyans were not convinced and remained very suspicious of the Rabbitskin leader's story. They still believed that their people were murdered by the Rabbitskin Nation. In a ploy to convince this group, Behzie suggested that they also make peace and exchange gifts.

Then people stood in a big line to exchange gifts. Behzie approached Ah Beh Cho with a whole moose hide and asked for the big knife that Ah Beh Cho was carrying on his belt. Ah Beh Cho said, "That moose hide looks pretty dry to me." But before Behzie had a chance to answer, a fight broke out at the end of the line. Suddenly, Ah Beh Cho pulled out his big knife and lunged at Behzie's belly.

Behzie was a very strong medicine-power person. In an instant, he spoke the elaborate verse that tells how steel was created. He said, "In the beginning all steel was liquid and I make it so again." The knife dripped onto the ground.

Ah Beh Cho fled in terror, but the warriors chased him down and killed him right there. All the warriors in the Chipewyan group were murdered that day. That was the last fight the Chipewyan people had with the Rabbitskin people.

29: Medicine Power and Hand Games

This is a story about a strong medicine man from Colville Lake. His name was Sah Yea Dene, which means "Inside the Sun Man." He played hand games with his people all his life. He was very good at it because he had medicine power for hand games. Inevitably, the side Sah Yea Dene played on won the game. All over the territory he was known for skill in hand games. Even when his opponents used medicine power against him, they were still unsuccessful. He was just too powerful. As you can imagine, it also made many people angry when he was unbeatable.

Hand games are simple games that Dene people have been playing for generations. The object of the game is to guess in which of his closed hands your opponent has placed a small item. You use your fingers to point to the hand that you believe has the object. Sticks are used to keep track of the score: there are four sticks per side if there is only one person on each side. More sticks are used for more players. It is possible to have up to thirty or forty players on each side. Each time you guess wrong, you must give your opponent one stick. The object can be moved into either hand after each unsuccessful guess. When you guess right, that person is knocked out of play. When all the players are knocked out of play, you switch sides and an opponent tries to guess which hand you, and your team players, have hidden the items.

The loser must pay the winner whatever they wagered at the beginning of the game. After the Dene had begun trading with the fur traders, it was common to play for small items like matches, plug tobacco, or shells. These days, they play for money.

Every spring when there is a gathering, a drum dance is planned that may last for many nights. The same is true for hand games. Sometimes, the games continue for three nights without sleep for the players.

It is tremendous fun! There are hand game songs that can be sung with or without the drum. The beat is quite lively and increases the excitement to a real frenzy. When there are ten to fifteen drums, they make quite a racket. To make it more interesting, people tease each other. Each person tries to outsmart the opponent who is trying to guess. It is interesting to watch the players because they are all different, and some people really have style. Taunting and teasing the other team is common.

When a good player is able to fool the opponent who is guessing, he really plays it up: yelling, shaking his empty hand at the other team, smiling, and acting real smug. The players often bounce to the beat of the drum as they wait for the opponent to decide which hand to guess. The tension while he is deciding is exhilarating.

The practice of playing hand games is an important aspect of Dene culture. With the poverty the Dene people have endured in the last two hundred years, it's understandable that the items that are wagered mean a great deal to the people who stand to lose them. With so much to lose, tempers are bound to rise, and players are tempted to take every advantage they can. Individuals have been known to use medicine power to prevent the opponent from guessing the right hand. Other people have used medicine power to help them guess.

Sah Yea Dene was one of those people. When the opponent chose his empty hand, he would whoop and move his arms and hands around to the beat of the drum. His long hair would be flying all around his head. He was a spectacle just to watch. He was always the last person left on his team because he was the best. Nobody could guess which hand held the item.

Around 1880 and 1890, trading for fur was good business in the north. Fort Good Hope was known as the best place for trading in the whole of the Mackenzie Valley. Colville Lake didn't have a store at that time, which meant the people from around Colville Lake would have to travel to Fort Good Hope to trade their furs. At Christmas, Easter, and in the spring, many people would gather in Fort Good Hope and hand games were always great entertainment.

It was during this time that Sah Yea Dene lived and was known for playing hand games. He was young then and a good hunter and trapper, and, of course, a superb hand games player.

This was the era of the Yukon's gold rush, which brought the 30-30 repeating rifle to the north. Prior to that, everybody was using the old muzzle-loading gun. Around 1890, the people from the Mackenzie River area travelled to the Yukon to buy the 30-30 repeating rifle. There was a huge crowd at Fort Good Hope that year, and many furs were sold there.

The trip to Whitehorse, Yukon, is approximately six hundred miles from Fort Good Hope. There were many people throughout the Yukon Territory who were strangers to the people from Fort Good Hope. When the group from Fort Good Hope got to Whitehorse, they quickly purchased the rifles and started off on their long journey home. It was a very long journey to get home, with many opportunities to meet new people along the way.

The Yukon Territory is home to Dene people as well. On their way home, the group came upon a village of Yukon Dene with whom they camped. As always, when Dene people gathered together, hand games were started. The group from Fort Good Hope played against the people from the Yukon village.

Sah Yea Dene was one of the players, and his team could not lose. The Yukon Dene were getting angry. They knew that Sah Yea Dene was using medicine power to help him win. The Yukon Dene tried to use different medicine-power men to guess which hand Sah Yea Dene's hid the object in, but they were still unsuccessful.

Sah Yea Dene is a great teaser, which is what infuriates his opponents. When they guess the wrong hand, he yells and makes a big fuss. After days of losing to Sah Yea Dene, and unbeknownst to the people from Fort Good Hope, the Yukon Dene sent for a very strong medicine-power person of their own. On the third night of hand games, the Yukon Dene's medicine man sat down in front of Sah Yea Dene and said, "Sah Yea Dene, just watch. I will guess right."

Sah Yea Dene just laughed and said, "I don't care." Other people had teased him before, but he still won.

At first, Sah Yea Dene was yelling and teasing like he always did. Then the medicine man clapped his hands together and pointed to Sah Yea Dene's hand. He was wrong: no object in his hand. But then something happened that no one expected. Suddenly, Sah Yea Dene's little finger fell to the ground. It was as if someone had cut it off with a knife. The crowd gasped and started to shout. Blood was spurting all over. They took the severed finger and burned it in the fire. Then they bandaged his hand. The hand games were over.

Shortly after, they resumed their journey home. When they reached their own community, the Elders had a meeting to discuss the trip to the Yukon and the incident with Sah Yea Dene. The Elders counselled him, "It is not good for you to travel too far from home again. You could start a medicine-power war and that would be bad for all the people. Many lives are lost in a war. Stay here with your relatives at Colville Lake where people know you well."

And this is what he did.

Another incident involving Sah Yea Dene took place close to Colville Lake. A group of people with about six dog teams was trapping on the Barren lands for white fox. They ran out of matches and shells and tea, so they headed for a small trading post at the north end of Great Bear Lake. There was a small village there. Again, they started to play hand games. As usual, Sah Yea Dene was winning.

After two nights of losing, the village Dene decided to ask for help from one of their medicine-power men, Dowyea. They sent someone to talk to him in his tent, where he was asleep.

They told him, "We have lost four hand games now and we owe them almost everything we own. Will you help us win it back?"

Dowyea agreed to play. He was known as a powerful medicine man. He was a Dogrib but spent all his life in the Great Bear Lake area. He sat down to play against Sah Yea Dene.

Abruptly, the tables were turned. No one could guess which hand hid Dowyea's object. The Yukon Dene were revived! They played and played until he won back all that they had lost. Then they played more, and he continued to win. Now it was the Fort Good Hope group's turn to be angry. Sah Yea Dene shouted, "Just you wait until it's my turn. I will take everything back. You'll never guess right on me."

But, of course, he would not get a turn until someone was able to guess right on Dowyea. Suddenly, Dowyea stood up. He said, "The game should stop."

He opened his hand to reveal a bullet. Dowyea said to them, "You will never get me. If we play for any longer, you will lose your dogs to us and then you will have to go home on foot. We will win everything you have. We are all Dene, and Dene people don't like to see each other suffer. I say we should stop the hand games now."

And that is what they did. That is the only time in his life that Sah

Yea Dene found a man equal to him in hand games.

That was a very strange situation. Usually, there are always medicine-power people around who have the ability to guess on the opposing player with great accuracy. But, in this case, there were none. The men that were playing had medicine power that gave them the ability to hide the object.

Sah Yea Dene explained that he received medicine power from the sun even before he was born. He described that time in this way: "Me and the sun talked to each other just like I talk to you. Before I was born, the sun and I played hand games with the moon and stars and other planets. It was such fun. Before we played, the sun gave me an object to play hand games with, and that is what I still use today. I have played hand games with this object all my life, and no one has ever guessed where it is hidden."

To explain further what Sah Yea Dene has said, I will offer this: when Sah Yea Dene says that he has played hand games in space with these planets, he means he has played with a spirit who represents each of these planets. The spirit takes on the form of a human with a personality, sense of humor, language, and other gifts. Sah Yea Dene played hand games with each of the spirits of the sun, moon, and other planets.

Sah Yea Dene was a difficult opponent to beat, both on Earth and in space. He lived on this Earth for one hundred and five years.

Dowyea never used medicine power to play before that incident. He only used it then because he could see that his people would lose everything they had to the Fort Good Hope group. He, too, was a strong medicine-power person. While he was asleep, he was actually using his gifts to investigate how Sah Yea Dene was wining without fail. He discovered that is was impossible to guess right when it came to Sah Yea Dene in a hand game.

A person would have to have the same kind of medicine power that Sah Yea Dene had in order to overcome him. Without this power, nothing could be done. But Dowyea also had received medicine power before he was born. One of his medicine gifts was something we call "living bullets." Dowyea could direct where a bullet goes just by thinking of the destination. This was a very useful gift for hunting; Dowyea always hit what he was shooting. He was a very successful hunter as a result.

Dowyea realized that if he used a bullet as the object in his hand during hand games, he could control it with his mind. He could make the bullet jump between his hands. When the opposing player guessed the object was in Dowyea's right hand, he would make it jump into his left hand, and so on. How could you guess against a person like that? You would have to have a person with equal medicine power that controls objects with the mind. At that time, there wasn't anyone there with that kind of power.

30: The Story of Bechachy

THIS IS A STORY ABOUT A CONFLICT INVOLVING TWO VERY STRONG medicine power men and the resulting loss of life. Bechachy was a man who lived his life in the area of Arctic Red River, which is now called Tsiigehtchic. Bechachy originally came from Fort Good Hope. Bechachy was a strong medicine-power person. At the time this incident happened, he was an old man with a son of about forty years old.

As one of the few English speaking Dene, Bechachy's son worked for the Hudson's Bay Company. He was a fur trader for the Company, but, by our people's standards, he was spoiled, proud, and a show off. He also had more material wealth than most of our people at the time, and he had no respect for Elders. Bechachy wouldn't listen to anyone! This, of course, is what got him into so much trouble.

The Hudson's Bay Company provided a big boat, similar to the rail boats, which Bechachy used to cross the Great Bear Lake. He often travelled far to find trappers and collect their furs. The Hudson's Bay Company also provided him with all the trade goods an Indian trapper needs in the bush. He exchanged the trade goods with the trappers for fur pelts. Sometimes, in the fall, a trapper was given supplies on credit with the understanding that the debt was payable in the spring after the winter season of trapping.

Still, as is the case with all groups of people, some Indians were poor and couldn't pay their debt when it came due, and others were dishonest and just plain refused to pay their debt. Bechachy's son was known for being mouthy and hard on anyone who did not pay their debts with him, regardless of the reason.

One spring, after a winter of travelling for the Hudson's Bay Company, Bechachy's son returned to Déline, which was called "Fort Franklin" at the time, to collect furs from people there. Many people were planning to travel to Fort Norman to trade their fur and buy the trade goods they needed. Bechachy's son was also keen to go and ensure anyone who had received credit from him last fall paid his or her debt.

One of the people who had a debt with the son was an Elder and a very strong medicine-power person named Bahwar. He owed sixty dollars. Bechachy's son approached Bahwar and demanded payment. Bahwar carefully explained his unfortunate situation.

Bahwar said, "This year I've had very tough luck. My daughter was sick throughout the winter and I was unable to trap. I know about my bill with you, but I have nothing to pay you. Just last week, I went into the bush with some people and they killed three beaver for me. We got one big, one medium, and one small beaver skin, which is all I have to buy tea and matches and live on all summer. I cannot give you any of the beaver skins to pay my debt. Don't worry, though: I will remember my bill next winter when I will trap again. Then I will pay you back."

One of the sacred laws that were taught to the people by Yamoria says, "Always show great respect for each other. Be careful to avoid hurting others with your actions and words. Always do good things for your people. Live in peace." This law is one of the instructions given to our people to help them live safely with each other and with people who possessed the powerful medicine power that existed at that time.

Bechachy's son said to Bahwar, "Old man, your troubles are of no concern to me. I will take your three beaver skins to cover your debt."

Bahwar pleaded with the son, "You cannot do this to me. I will suffer all summer without these few furs to trade." But the son ignored him. He told him, "You are poor, but it is not my fault. You have to pay your bill like anyone else."

So Bahwar tried again: "I will make a deal with you then. I have six pups. They will be good dogs and just right for next winter. You can pick out the best two dogs to cover my bill with you."

Then the son got angry and shouted, "I don't want dogs! I want the three beaver skins, and that's what I'm going to take. You think that just because you have medicine power you can do whatever you want. You think people are scared of you. Well, I'm not! I'm a medicine man and my father is a very powerful medicine man." Then he screamed, "We're not scared of anyone!"

By this time, Bahwar was angry. When a medicine man becomes very angry, such as Bahwar was, his medicine power responds to his feelings and becomes instantly activated.

Bahwar stood up and commanded the son, "Get out of my tent! I don't want to see you again for as long as I live. I will never pay my bill with you now, and you won't get my dogs either. You won't need them where you're going anyhow!"

Now, for the first time, the man felt afraid. He scrambled out of the old man's tent without saying another word. By October of the same year the son was dead. People had heard the loud dispute between the two men, including Bahwar's threat. When the son died in October, gossip spread quickly that Bahwar killed a man with medicine power.

By Christmas of the same year, the news reached Fort Good Hope and Bechachy. They said his son was dead. He also heard the story that Bahwar killed his son with medicine power. Troubled by the events of his son's death, Bechachy made up his mind that he would travel to Fort Norman in the spring to see what he could find out.

Spring was a busy time. Trappers gathered at the trading posts to exchange their furs for supplies. Fort Norman was an important trading post and many Dene people gathered from miles around to trade and visit. In summer, there are several drum dances, feasts, and hand games competitions. At one of these feasts near Fort Norman, an unfortunate event happened.

After hours of preparation, the food for the feast was ready. However, before every feast, leaders take the opportunity to first speak to the people. In this group, there were four chiefs and several other community leaders. For over an hour they each took their turn addressing the crowd. Finally, they were ready to say a prayer and then food would be eaten.

Suddenly, an old man started to yell, "I have something I want to say!"

The chief answered him, "If you have something to say, make it real short. The people are hungry! And can you introduce yourself so we will know who you are!"

In the language of the people from Fort Good Hope he said, "My name is Bechachy. I come from the other side of Fort Good Hope, about fifty miles this side of Arctic Red River. I come from a long way. I came here to see someone in particular. I want you people to know about it. As soon as the Mackenzie River broke, I put my wife in the canoe and paddled up the river all the way here. That is four hundred miles. I just arrived here during the night. I slept on the shore down here. Thank you. I will eat with you people, but first I will tell you why I came here. You see, I am not a person who believes in gossiping. I don't talk behind anyone's back. When there's a problem, I like to talk directly to the person responsible. And that's what I'm here to do.

"Last summer, my oldest son, who worked for the Hudson's Bay

Company, travelled all over the Great Bear Lake for his work. You know, I really love my son, but he died in Fort Norman last fall. I heard something about his death that is heavy on my heart. This is what I'm here to investigate. I was told that my son was killed with medicine power by a person by the name of Bahwar."

The crowd was silent. Bechachy continued, "If this person, Bahwar, is here in this crowd, let him identify himself."

Now Bahwar was the strongest medicine power person alive at that time. With the confidence of a man who controls a terrific power, Bahwar, stood up to face Bechachy. He spoke calmly and without fear: "My name is Bahwar. If you are talking about me and want to talk to me, well, then here I am, my friend. I am listening."

Bechachy asked, "It is true that you killed my son? I want to hear it from you."

Bahwar paused for a moment, then looked up at Bechachy and said simply, "Yes, it's true." Then he continued, "It is also true that your son caused his own death. Your son was a rough man to deal with. He had a big mouth, which is what got him into trouble. You know, when the world was new, the great Yamoria established laws that all people should follow. It is the responsibility of all parents to teach their children about these laws. Now I see that, as a parent, you did not teach your son too well. You spoiled him instead. I did not know your son very well, but still he came to me demanding that I pay him sixty dollars.

"If your son listened to the laws, as taught by Yamoria, he would be alive today. Instead, he talked himself into an early grave. From the way I see it, you are also responsible for your son's death."

As Bahwar spoke, Bechachy grew more and more angry. Finally, when he was burning with rage, he roared, "If you like to kill people, then try me! At least I am a real man!"

The crowd was very alarmed to hear talk of killing. "Please stop it. Don't talk like that!" someone shouted.

But the two medicine men had no intention of stopping. They

continued to shout and throw threats at each other. Bechachy said, "Now we are going to kill each other, but I tell you one thing for sure: I won't be the first to go. You, old man, will die first."

Bahwar spit, "If you kill me, I will take all your medicine people with me."

By now the crowd was talking all at once. Some were crying. They knew the strong medicine power that existed here and feared disaster would result from all this anger and the threats. They begged them to stop. Finally, they found another medicine man who went up to each of them and hit the top of their heads with his hat. Then he blew over their heads. Finally, they stopped.

The chief tried to take control of the situation. He said, "It's too bad this had to happen here. This was supposed to be a happy occasion, but we are not happy now. Please, if you cannot eat here now, take the food home and eat it there."

In despair, the crowd dispersed to eat with their families.

This was the beginning of great tragedy among Dene people of the north. People hoped that everything would be alright. They hoped that the incident was just a quarrel between two old men. But, by the morning of the third day, their hopes were shattered. Bahwar died. Then, before sunset, Bechachy died. After that, a great sickness came upon the people. Many second-class medicine people followed Bahwar and Bechachy to the spirit world. Then Elders, who had only a few items of medicine power, died.

Only the young, without medicine power, survived at first. Still, the sickness was not the only problem. Starvation was soon to follow. With so many people ill, there was no one left to find food. At that time the store only sold dry goods, like flour and rolled oats, but no meat. In Fort Norman there were no fish whatsoever.

Only five years before, in 1921, the people had signed a treaty that guaranteed help from the government in times of sickness and famine. However, no help came.

What did come were the rains. It rained and wouldn't stop until the Mackenzie River overflowed its banks. Still, the people were too ill to look after what they owned. Canoes were lost. Dogs tied on the shore drowned.

Many trappers and their families, people of the Great Bear Lake area, were at the trading post at the time. Half of them never made it back home but perished in the epidemic. The people from the Mackenzie River moved away from town to escape peril. This incident was a great tragedy for Dene people that Elders still talk about today.

As you can see from this story, the ownership of medicine power is a grave responsibility. The Elders teach us to always keep your mind, body, emotions, and spirit in balance with each other. They also say to control your anger toward others. When a person owns medicine power, he or she becomes a partner with the spirit of that medicine power. Then they communicate with each other and work together.

In the case of Bahwar and Bechachy, they possessed more medicine power than most people at the time—perhaps up to three hundred different items of medicine power. When they allowed themselves to get in such a rage, they triggered the medicine power they possessed. It's as if the spirit of the medicine power was awakened into a similar rage. Then the energy behind the rage was directed toward the object of their anger, which, in this case, was each other and other medicine-power people.

When you wake up such an angry force of medicine power, the way these two men did, it is impossible to contain. This is why the two medicine men were unable to stop once they started to quarrel with such fury.

Still, in my opinion, it was a criminal act for Bahwar to say he would take all the other medicine-power people with him in death. He also created the sickness in the north, and many, many people suffered and perished all over the Northwest Territories because of his recklessness.

Today, the disaster of 1926 is still talked about by many Elders in the north. Dene people have suffered ever since relying on the government for many things. Truly, we have never recovered from this devastation. Since that summer, we have never seen the strength in medicine power within our people that was present at that time.

In my opinion, if ever a person deserved to be punished for their crimes with medicine power, it was these two men, Bahwar and Bechachy. Unfortunately, Dene people do not have a system of justice to punish people who commit crimes with medicine power. The only retribution that I have ever heard of occurs when a relative of the person who was murdered seeks out a medicine person and then hires them to use their medicine power to attack the person who murdered their relative. Usually, though, nothing is ever done about these crimes.

Can you imagine living in a community with a medicine person who has murdered people with their medicine power—and knowing about it? Understandably, most people are too afraid to ever confront them.

31: The Story of Gotaregai

THIS IS A VERY OLD STORY ABOUT A FIRST-CLASS MEDICINE-POWER person by the name of Gotaregai. He spent all his life in the mountain range, living among the Aboriginal people of the area. Gotaregai was a feared man because of his reputation for using medicine power to commit crimes and violence. Most people tried to stay out of his way lest they become the victim of one of his acts of violence.

One year, Gotaregai, his sister, and her husband were travelling alone to harvest food from the land. They were very successful and killed many big game animals. They made dry meat and then constructed a cage to store it in until they would need it in the winter. Then they moved on to continue to hunt and harvest the land. They travelled continuously until winter.

When winter came, they set off to look for the dry meat they had put away. It seemed that a late frost on the trees had changed the look of the countryside, and Gotaregai's brother-in-law had a very difficult time locating the stash. He searched and searched until he was completely lost and confused.

Gotaregai became very angry with his brother-in-law. In a rage, he picked up a club and smashed his head in. The man died right there. Still, Gotaregai and his sister continued to travel on the land until they came to a big lake. They noticed, across the shore, a fish camp with many, many people living there. The group had nets set under the ice.

Without being noticed, Gotaregai watched the group a long while. He believed all people hated him, and it pained him greatly. He wondered to himself, "If I were a baby, would these people still hate me, or, instead, would they take care of me and look after me with love?" He decided to find out what the group would do.

Suddenly, Gotaregai changed himself into a baby. Wearing nothing but a makeshift diaper and bare feet, he crawled over to the group. At first they didn't know what this was crawling on the ground. Then they thought it was a small animal. Finally, when the baby got close enough, they realized what they were looking at. They were astounded.

"What is a baby doing on the ice in the middle of winter?" someone asked. Then he suggested, "Let's chase it!" Another person grabbed a club and lunged at the baby. The baby quickly moved out of the way. Try as they might, they could not get ahold of the baby. Finally, they surrounded the baby and attempted to jump on him and grab him. Still, the baby crawled through their legs and escaped. At last they gave up.

By this time, Gotaregai realized that these people would not take pity on him even if he was a small baby. Surely, they would have killed him if they could have caught him. Feelings of contempt and hatred boiled up within him. With great malice, he imagined how he would teach them a lesson and inflict his revenge. Then, in an instant, Gotaregai transformed from a toddler into a giant of a man. In terror, the people shrieked, "It's Gotaregai!" and ran blindly in all directions. Gotaregai hunted each one down and clubbed them to death.

When the massacre had ended, Gotaregai and his sister once again continued to travel on the land. Only now, the weight of Gotaregai's crimes burdened him. Awake or asleep, bloody images and screaming voices haunted him. Gotaregai knew that he, alone, had not done this; he understood that his feelings of hatred had triggered the fury of the medicine power he possessed. Together they had carried out his evil fantasies. He felt very sorry for himself.

By now, hatred had also grown within Gotaregai's sister. She had witnessed his evil acts and felt tremendous loss with the death of her husband, the only man she had ever loved. She began to fantasize how she would avenge her husband's murder. Then she devised a plot.

One morning, she awoke early before Gotaregai. She got up, built a fire, and started to cook. She listened intently to Gotaregai's snoring—breathing in, then breathing out. Then, suddenly, she decided that now was her chance. She quietly reached for the club and raised it to smash his head. It was the last thing she ever did. Gotaregai's medicine power, even when he was asleep, protected him. In less than a heartbeat, he grabbed the club from her hand and smashed her head into the ground.

Now he was truly alone and miserable. He travelled and travelled. He was in the greatest distress he had ever known. He thought about killing himself but decided that he could not do it. He travelled southeast and followed the big mountain range. After a long journey he reached the ocean.

Here he found a village of people who lived by harvesting the sea. He stayed with them for a time and was very careful to stay out of trouble and not harm anyone. These people had never heard of Gotaregai and his crimes and, therefore, accepted him with trust and respect. But Gotaregai could not rest. His past tormented his mind. He sought relief from his anguish. He decided to tell the Elders the truth about his past and beg for their help.

Gotaregai told them the stories of his crimes. When he was done he addressed the people: "I have killed everybody around me for no reason. It's true. I have done these useless things. Now they are all gone, and I am here without my family, without my people, without anything but suffering.

"You do not need to be afraid of me, though. I will not harm anyone here. I have no mind for that anymore. All I can think of is my own suffering. I want to die. I want to join my people in the spirit world. I desperately need your help. Will you take pity on a suffering man? I'm asking you to kill me. I know it's not an easy proposition. I'm begging for your help!"

At first the group wanted no part in this killing of Gotaregai. But he was so pitiful that he would not give up. Finally, an Elder asked, "What if we threw him in that bad lake? Surely those big insects would eat him up in no time."

When Gotaregai heard this he was relentless. He pleaded for them to end his misery by throwing him in the lake. Then it was decided: they would help.

The entire village packed up and travelled to the lake. They would all stand witness to this act. They reassured Gotaregai, "We will throw you in this lake and in no time you will be dead."

Gotaregai replied, "Yes, do it."

So a group grabbed Gotaregai and threw him off the bank and into the lake. The entire village stood and witnessed what they believed would be the last of that pitiful medicine-power man. Before they had time to disperse, a ghost of a man walked out from the depths of the lake onto the shore.

It was an eerie sight, and they ran for the bushes in horror. A few Elders stood and waited for Gotaregai to approach them. He was nothing but bones and rags. He spoke: "Look for something sharp and pierce the thing I am holding in my fist. It is my heart. Yes, it is in the middle of my hand. I am not the same as other people."

As the Elder pierced his hand, blood began to spray from the wound. Then, in a crumpled heap, the body fell to the ground. Finally, that was the end Gotaregai's life on Mother Earth. Everywhere he went, people were scared of him and never got close to him. He lived a wicked but tormented and lonely life.

It would be good to try to understand Gotaregai's life from the perspective of medicine power. It's true he was a powerful medicine-power person. In the beginning, he didn't intend on becoming a criminal. But, as time passed, he got mixed up with other medicine-power people who eventually tried to kill him with medicine power. He was very young at the time and was compelled to fight for his life. His medicine power helped him to escape the wrath of these evil medicine-power men.

Still, that experience transformed Gotaregai into a bitter and violent man who had an uncontrollable temper that got worse as he got older. Elders say that when Gotaregai was young he cured people when they got sick. They say he had medicine power over the human body. It was very easy for him to heal a person. He could have become one of the greatest healers of his people, but, after he started into a life of violence, he didn't care to heal people anymore. Gotaregai could have done great acts of good for all people. Instead, he is remembered for the great acts of evil he committed.

32: The Story of Edzo

WHEN THE WORLD WAS NEW, ABORIGINAL PEOPLE TRAVELLED A GREAT deal across this immense land. We harvested the land, not only to provide food for ourselves but to acquire hides for clothing. The anthropologists say we were nomadic, which means that we never stayed in one place but moved around steady.

Medicine power was an integral part of the governance of our nations at that time. Most Dene leaders were also medicine-power people because they possessed gifts that allowed them to do things that the average person could not. Also, many people were in awe and even afraid of their medicine people and, therefore, listened when they gave advice. Edzo was such a person. Edzo was a first-class medicine person from the Dogrib Nation. He lived among his own people all his life, and there are many stories told about this remarkable man.

He was a great leader and powerful medicine man. He led with a strong voice and his people followed him willingly. His reputation was known far and wide. When Edzo was alive, the fur traders were just starting to come north. They had only reached the borders of Alberta, British Columbia, and Saskatchewan and, therefore, the tribes north of these areas did not have access to luxuries such as axes, knives, and matches. Only the biggest of nations had enough furs to attract the fur traders into their area.

Still, Edzo was determined to acquire the wares of the fur traders. However, he had one big problem that prevented him from doing this easily: the Chipewyan Nation. Relations between the two nations were strained at best. The Dogrib people could expect trouble if they tried to travel deep into Chipewyan territory to find the fur traders.

When Edzo heard that the fur traders were near the British Columbia and Northwest Territories border, he decided to travel into that area to find them. Ten families travelled with him on the flat lands near the Mackenzie River. They crossed the river below Fort Simpson and then headed south, deep into the Rocky Mountains. In late winter, he sent two men farther south to find the fur traders. They waited and waited for the men to return, but they were never seen again. Edzo was puzzled by this and so sent two more men south to find the fur traders, or the first two men, or both. They waited all through spring and then summer, but the second pair never returned.

When winter came again, Edzo told his people, "We are strangers in this country and too far away from our own territory and our own people. It is dangerous to stay here much longer. Our presence here could start a war. I think it is best if we return to our own lands." Soon after, the people made the journey back home. They crossed the Mackenzie River easily because it was still winter and the river was frozen, then headed toward the bush country near Hollow Lake.

It was springtime when they finally reached their own home territory. Here they joined one of the many groups that were camped in the area between Hollow Lake and Fort Rae. There was a large population of Dogrib people in this area. For them, it was customary to travel to the Barren lands each summer to hunt caribou.

At that time, the Chipewyan Nation was the largest tribe in the north. They hunted caribou on the Barren lands much like the Dogrib Nation. This year, everyone was talking about the Chipewyan Nation. Apparently, the Chipewyan people were threatening war against the Dogrib people. Some Chipewyan hunters had gone out and never returned. They believed Dogrib people were responsible. Their leader was telling everyone, "If we catch any of those Dogribs on the Barren lands, we're going to kill them dead!"

This was very bad news. The Chipewyan Nation was a powerful force. They had three times the population of the Dogrib Nation and were known for their strength in medicine power. Their leader, Akaitcho, was a formidable medicine man. The Dogrib people faced a great dilemma. If they hunted for the precious caribou in the Barren lands, they may be attacked and killed by the Chipewyan. If they didn't hunt for caribou, they would surely starve this winter without any meat.

As the time to hunt caribou grew close, the people grew more distressed. A great meeting was organized to discuss their situation and decide what would be done. There were many speeches that cautioned against provoking the Chipewyan Nation. The fear was tangible.

Then, when it seemed everyone had spoken, Edzo, who had been sitting quietly, stood up. He said, "I am not afraid of the Chipewyans. I am not afraid of anyone. It has always been our custom to hunt caribou on the Barren lands each summer. We do this because it is how we survive. It is our way. We cannot miss a hunt because we are afraid of someone. Then what kind of people would we be? I will go onto the Barren lands to hunt. Perhaps I will find their great leader there, Akaitcho. I will convince him that the Dogrib Nation wants peace. I ask for ten men to travel with me."

But the fear was great, and no one volunteered to accompany Edzo. Finally, a young boy of fifteen, Edzo's nephew, said, "I'll go with you, Uncle." Then Edzo looked right at his brother-in-law, who was also a strong medicine man. "Are you with me, my brother?"

"I am," he answered.

They left as soon as they could pack the things they would need.

Many nights later they reached the Barren lands. They became very alert, searching for signs that the Chipewyan people were near. They climbed to the top of a hill and saw in the distance a camp with many tents. They had found the Chipewyan Nation. As it was late in the day, they made camp by a small bunch of trees and unpacked some dry meat to eat.

Edzo turned and said, "Wait here. I want to get a closer look. My sister is married to a Chipewyan. If I can find her, she could be a big help to us. I will be back before daylight."

Secretly, Edzo made his way to the big camp. When he got close enough, he found a trail that the people used to get water. There he found a hiding place and waited quietly. His one hope was that his sister would pass by on her way to get water and he would be able to talk to her alone. He waited only a short time when he heard someone walking down the path. He hid himself carefully and watched the trail. His heart leaped when he saw that it was, in fact, his sister. He stepped quickly in front of her and motioned for her to be quiet.

Edzo's sister whispered to him, "Come with me before anyone sees you!" Then she led him to her tent and ducked inside. Only when she secured the door did she allow herself to smile at him. Then she said to him, "Let's fix a place for you to hide just in case someone comes in. My husband is at the gathering place with the rest of them. Every day they go there and talk about the Dogrib people. They say the Dogrib people killed the hunters that never returned. Akaitcho has promised to kill any Dogrib found in the territory. Please, my brother, go back home. Do not stay here!"

Just then, her husband came into the tent. Although surprised to see Edzo in his tent he soon was telling him the same thing: "You are better off if you head home right away. People are angry, and it is dangerous here for even you, Edzo."

But Edzo was a stubborn man. He had to find a way to speak with Akaitcho. He told them, "As you know, I cannot go home without speaking to Akaitcho or our people will starve this winter without any caribou. I have a plan, but I will need your help. Tomorrow morning, take some men with you and go hunting on the shore of the big lake. I will make camp in an open spot where you are sure to see us as you come around the point in your canoes. When you see our camp you can persuade the men to come back here and tell Akaitcho there are Dogribs in your territory. I will wait for you all to return with Akaitcho. He will come to me and then I will be able to speak to him."

When Edzo got back to his camp, he ate with the two men and explained what had happened. Then, early in the morning, they moved their camp near the shore where they were sure to be seen by travellers in the water. He told his brother in law, "I know you have power for mind control. You will have to use it the best you can to stop them from killing us."

Edzo's brother in law took out a beaver hide and heated it up on the fire. When it became soft, he told Edzo, "I will make medicine power

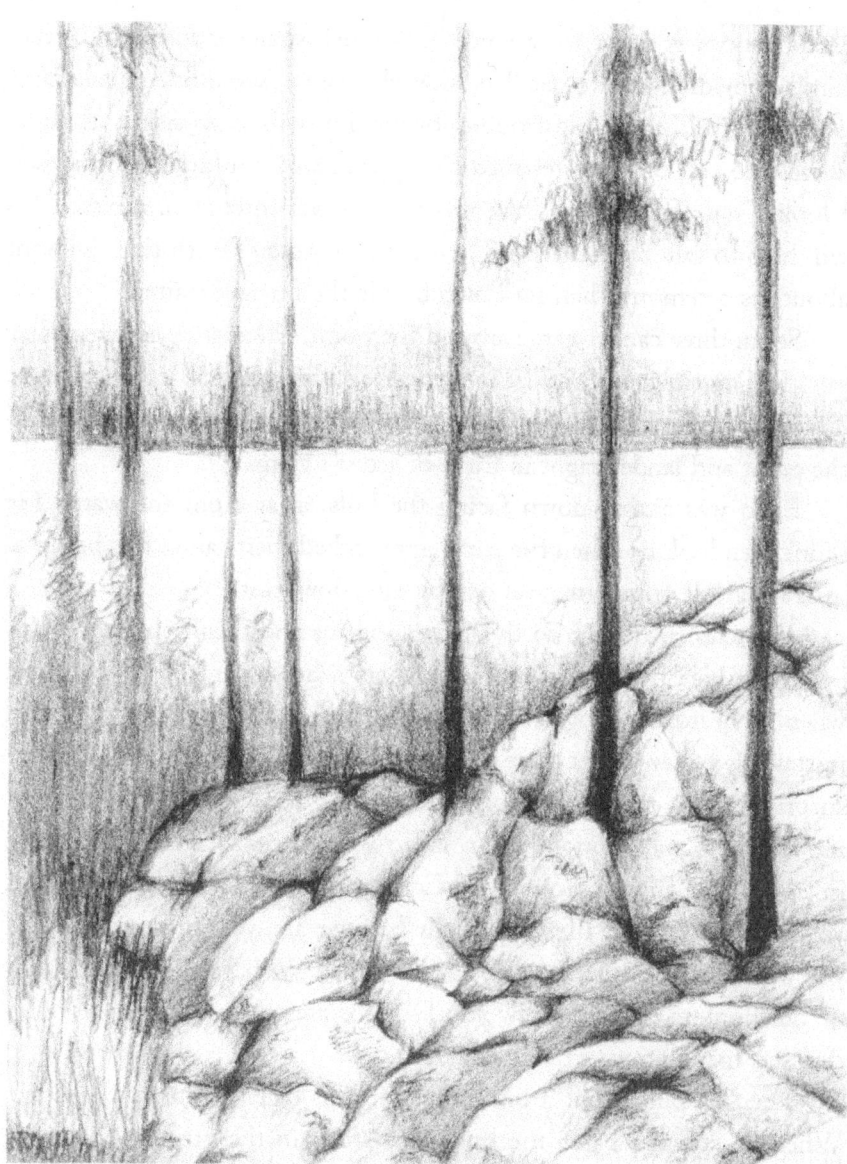

now. I will put all their thinking in the beaver hide. Then I will sit on it and control their minds. They can do as they like, but I will make them think what I want them to think." He finished his ceremony and then sat on the beaver hide.

Then Edzo began to make medicine power. "I will call on the

medicine-power spirit for a voice. It is much stronger than most other kinds of medicine power. Still, if Akaitcho has the same kind of medicine power, it could mean big trouble for me. I'm willing to risk it, though. I will also call on monster medicine power that could change the way I look. Then, finally, I will use medicine power to control minds. This will help to talk to Akaitcho. Then I will be ready." With that, he went about his ceremony, then sat down beside the fire and waited.

Soon, three canoes came around the point. They stopped when they saw the Dogrib camp, and Edzo could hear the sound of excited voices. Then they turned back. Not long afterward, many canoes came around the point and landed right in front of Edzo's camp.

Edzo was sitting down facing the hills, away from the water. He didn't even look up when the party approached their camp. His brother-in-law and the young man sat nearby, eyes downcast.

Akaitcho rushed up to the three Dogribs and then paused. He was breathing hard. Akaitcho was a big man who had raced to get there when he heard the Dogrib men were in their territory. The group had mistakenly believed that there was a large group of Dogrib and were very surprised to see these three docile men sitting alone by the fire.

Akaitcho walked right up to Edzo where he was sitting and spoke in a booming, angry voice, "Well, Edzo, it is you! I have wanted to meet you in person all my life, and finally here we are, you and me. Too bad you will also be the first Dogrib I will ever kill. We have been losing many of our hunters, and we know you Dogribs are to blame. Every Dogrib that sets foot in our territory is a dead one."

Then he pulled out a big knife from his belt and lunged at Edzo. When he stepped back, the knife was stuck in the ground up to the handle, and Edzo was sitting calm and still, facing the hills, head down. Edzo's calm, in spite of Akaitcho's attempts to provoke him, puzzled all the Chipewyans, especially Akaitcho. It wasn't what he expected, and he seemed unsure of what to do next.

Then, slowly, Edzo brought himself to a standing position and turned to face his attacker. A gasp was audible from the crowd as Edzo looked up for the first time and they caught sight of his face. He was ugly beyond belief. His long hair was wet with sweat and his eyes were black and shiny like glass. He was drooling from both sides of his mouth. He looked fierce and dangerous and angry all at the same time.

Just then, a black cloud blew in above them, lightning flashed, and a clap of thunder followed. The wind blew the small willows until their tops touched the ground. A booming voice rang out, "You are going to kill me? You are going to kill every Dogrib?" Then Edzo roared, "Well then, what are you waiting for?" The wind seemed to rage in response to his words and blew even stronger.

The Chipewyans were visibly shaken. Even Akaitcho had a shocked look on his face. This wasn't anything like what they had anticipated. They stood facing Edzo, dumbfounded, their eyes fixed on his hideous face.

Then the wind subsided and the sun came out again. Edzo spoke, "Maybe you want to make peace instead? Maybe you want to make peace with your neighbours, us pitiful Dogribs. Isn't that right, Akaitcho?"

It took a moment for Akaitcho to realize that this creature in front of him wanted an answer. At first he stammered, "Yes, yes, that's right." Then he seemed to recover and said, "If we kill each other here today a great war will be started that may never end. Mothers will be crying in our camps for a long, long time. Peace is always the best way. It is what the Chipewyan people want. It is what we have always wanted, Edzo."

Edzo regarded Akaitcho sternly. He replied, "Well, let us talk peace, then. From this day forward no one—not Dogrib nor Chipewyan—will be permitted to kill one another. If this law is broken, it will be the duty of the people to report this act to the leaders. Then the murderer will be put to death. This is a serious thing I am saying. We will not allow murderers to live among us. It will be up to each nation to enforce this law. This is the peace that I am talking about. Is this the kind of peace that you want?" His appearance softened in the sunlight. He continued, "Yamoria taught that we should love each other as much as possible and never harm another person. If we follow this teaching we will no longer have these problems. He also taught that we are to live as brothers and sisters on Mother Earth. This is the peace that we Dogrib people want." Edzo stood before them, the beast that had challenged them was transformed.

Then Akaitcho spoke, "I agree with all you have said." Akaitcho reached out to shake hands with his new ally. Then Akaitcho shouted so everyone could here, "Edzo and his relatives will come to our camp. We will gather the people together and tell them about this new peace treaty that we have agreed to here today. Then it will be time to celebrate. We will have a feast!"

The three Dogrib men followed Akaitcho to the large camp. The Chipewyans were puzzled to see their leader bringing Dogribs into their camp in such a peaceful fashion. In a short time the whole camp was gathered together waiting to hear what they had to say. Akaitcho asked Edzo to repeat the peace treaty for all who were listening. Then he got up and said, "I agree with Edzo. This is what we want: a peaceful life between our nations. And so it shall be! Now we must work on building friendly relationships with each other. Then the violence will be forgotten forever."

The whole camp stood in line and shook hands with each of the Dogrib men and with each other. Then preparations for the feast were made and a tea dance followed. They had such a good time that the celebration lasted for two days and nights. This is how peace was established between the two nations.

DEFINING MEDICINE POWER

This is a story of two powerful leaders and medicine men: Akaitcho and Edzo. This is also a story of one man underestimating his opponent. Akaitcho had never met Edzo before, but he knew about him from the many stories that were told throughout the country. He knew of his strength with medicine power. Still, when he heard that Edzo was camped on the shore of the lake, he rushed out to challenge him. This was a mistake. If he had investigated with his medicine power, he would have known what to expect. Instead, he was caught off guard and this gave Edzo an advantage. Akaitcho attempted to use medicine power on Edzo when he first approached him, but it was useless because Edzo was prepared for him.

Edzo had time and a plan. He had already done an investigation with his medicine power. He also had the help of his brother-in-law. Between the two of them, their combined medicine power to control the Chipewyan men's minds was unbeatable. In this case, they used their medicine power for a very valuable reason. They made the whole nation eager to accept peace. This is because Edzo and his brother were thinking for them.

Edzo used monster medicine power to change his appearance and scare the Chipewyan men. He used medicine power over the elements to make the wind blow and the thunder and lightning crash, which was also frightening. The voice of the medicine power spirit bellowing out of Edzo's mouth was unsettling to hear. All these things combined were a powerful force used to turn what could have been a tragedy into a positive page in Dene history.

33: THE RABBITSKIN PEOPLE

AT ONE TIME, A GROUP OF RABBITSKIN PEOPLE WAS LIVING NEAR A lake where they could fish all year round. They didn't travel far because it was a time of war and enemy tribes were near. Still, there was another fish lake about ten miles away where they also liked to set their fishnets. One day, four fishermen travelled to the next fish lake.

Among the Rabbitskin people lived a poor widow with a son of fifteen. Her son was known to possess medicine power and was very capable of taking care of his mother. He hunted chickens and ptarmigan along with fishing, and he kept them both well fed. Then, while the four fishermen were away at the next fish lake, the boy received a message from the spirit of his medicine power warning him that the enemy was near and a fight would soon result.

The boy thought to himself, "What will I do to escape when the enemy comes?" Then he had an idea. First, he dug a big hole in the deep snow behind their tent. Then, every time he killed a ptarmigan, he put the feathers in the hole. His plan was to jump in the hole and cover himself with feathers when the enemy came.

Nearby, a group of Chipewyan warriors were looking for the Rabbitskin people to attack them. They were travelling fast and late into the night. The Elder that was with them could not keep up. Instead, he took his time and followed their trail. One night, the Elder was resting when he smelled smoke as if from a campfire. He quietly investigated but found nothing. He thought to himself, "Maybe we missed a camp of Rabbitskin people." Later, he caught up with his people who were camped for the night and told them about the smell of smoke.

They sent out two men that night to search the area. When the men returned they reported that a group of Rabbitskin people was camping at the fish lake. Immediately they planned an attack. The warriors silently crept nearer to the camp and waited for the first sign of light. Then, before the sun crept over the horizon, they ran into camp with their spears and stabbed the people still asleep in their tents.

The widow's son heard the noise, tore off his blanket, and jumped in the hole full of ptarmigan feathers to hide. After what seemed a long time it was quiet again. He cautiously emerged from the hole and looked around to make sure no one was there. Still, it was not completely daylight yet. He quickly grabbed his snowshoes and snuck away. He ran as fast as he could to the lake and followed a trail to the next fish lake where the men had gone the day before.

Finally, out of breath and sweating, he reached the men. "Save yourselves!" he shouted. "The Chipewyan's have attacked our people! They will soon find you too."

The men all looked at each other. "What we need is medicine power," one said. "There's no time to waste. Look! Here they come now across the lake!"

Sure enough, the Chipewyans were paddling fast toward them.

The medicine man shouted, "I have medicine power for twist wind. All of you come here. Push that burning wood aside. Put some spruce branches where the fire has warmed the ground. We will all sit together, cover ourselves with a blanket, and hold onto each other." Then he began his medicine power ceremony. As he recited the complicated wording, a black cloud suddenly appeared in the sky. The wind picked up and began to blow harder and harder. Soon, they were covered with drifted snow.

They didn't move and were soon fast asleep. They slept and slept for two days. Finally, the medicine man woke them up. They dug themselves out of the hole, but what they found was a shock. The land they knew so well was changed. Trees were broken everywhere, and the snow was drifted higher than any of them had ever seen.

They made fire, had a meal of fish, and talked about their good fortune to be alive after such a close shave with death. In time, they travelled back to where their relatives lived on the shore of the main fish lake. We'll never know exactly what happened to the Chipewyan warriors. The twist wind is a powerful force.

34: THE RABBITSKIN AND CHIPEWYAN NATIONS AT WAR

IT'S COMMON KNOWLEDGE THAT THERE WERE MANY WARS BETWEEN different Aboriginal nations. But what you may not know is that, in many cases, the Dene in conflict began using medicine power. Sometimes a person is murdered using medicine power and the relatives of that person take revenge. Then a medicine war begins.

You see, with medicine power, a person could be attacked even though the aggressor is a thousand miles away. Then another medicine person could perform a ceremony to identify the aggressor. This is what happened once between the Chipewyan and Rabbitskin Nations. Once, a Rabbitskin person murdered a Chipewyan with medicine power. Then, in retaliation, a Chipewyan person murdered a Rabbitskin person with medicine power. This caused a great hatred between the two tribes.

Then, later that year, in December, the lake was frozen and travel was good. A small group of young and strong Chipewyan warriors travelled ahead of their tribe. They knew the area well and hunted as they travelled. They stopped to set fishnets and catch trout and other kinds of fish for drying. They knew they would need a good supply for the long journey ahead.

Behind them followed the women, children, and Elders. They were slower and were responsible for pulling the toboggans. These sleds were made of caribou leg hide and shaped like a long sack. In them, families would pool their belongings and this worked very well.

At the same time, a Rabbitskin tribe was hunting, fishing, and travelling in the area. However, their system of travel was very different than the Chipewyans'. The Rabbitskin group chose a slower pace so that the whole group could travel together. No one was left behind. They didn't know it, but each group was headed toward the other.

One day, as the Rabbitskin group was heading around a point of trees that grew on a spit of land that jutted far into the lake, they happened upon the group of Chipewyan warriors. There was no turning back or hiding. Both groups saw each other at the same time. The Chipewyan warriors took up their weapons and ran toward the Rabbitskin people. The Rabbitskin group faced the warriors and fought for their lives.

The battle went on and on until there were only two people left alive. One was the leader and a strong medicine man from the Rabbitskin tribe. The other was the leader and a strong medicine man from the Chipewyan tribe. Those two men fought and fought, but try as they did, they could not kill each other. They even rested and then fought again, but with their medicine power to protect each of them, their opponent could not win. They were equal in medicine-power strength.

Finally, they sat silently facing each other, exhausted. After a long silence the Chipewyan man spoke: "You are one tough man! Our women and Elders will be coming soon. They were travelling behind us. Why don't we make fire and eat?"

The Rabbitskin man agreed, so they sat together and cooked fish. After a time, the Chipewyan group arrived. It was a strange sight to see these two men sitting quietly together eating fish. The lake was a bloody battleground littered with the dead bodies of all those who had fallen.

The Chipewyan leader spoke to the group, "As you can see, a terrible battle has happened here today. We are the only survivors, although we have fought each other for many hours."

Just then an old man yelled in a rage, "My sons! All my sons are dead! What are you doing? Kill this Rabbitskin garbage. If you won't, I will!"

The Chipewyan leader answered, "Quiet, old man, if you want to live!" Then he turned to the people. "We will have to go back. There is nothing to continue on for anymore."

To the Rabbitskin leader he said, "You have nothing now. Your wife and children are lost. You might as well come with us. I will look after you. Perhaps in time you will find a good wife here with us. The Rabbitskin leader accepted and joined the Chipewyan tribe.

35: The Story of Sahlie

THIS IS THE STORY OF SAHLIE, WHO WAS A MEDICINE MAN WHO received all his medicine power before he was born—what I call a "first-class medicine person." The name *Sahlie* translates to "the nerve of the sun." As you may have guessed, Sahlie had medicine power for the sun, including all items related to how it exists today and how it was created. This is an unusual kind of medicine power to have, although we do know of others who had sun medicine power. Still, none had sun medicine power to the extent of Sahlie.

The stories of Sahlie have been told many times by Dene storytellers, which makes him quite famous to my people. Sahlie explained how he received medicine power: "The sun spirit came to me in a vision when I was a small child. He took the form of a man and said to me, 'I am the sun. We will work together in the future. Always remember that if you ever need my help, just call on me and I will be there.'"

As a child, and later as a teenager, Sahlie practiced ways to use his medicine power. Once when Sahlie was just a child, he noticed sunlight shining through a hole in the tent. He reached out to touch it and was shocked to find that it was hard and hot. This surprised him and he called out in fear. In an instant the sun spirit was there. "What's the problem, little one?" asked the sun spirit. "You don't need to be afraid."

Sahlie felt better that his friend was there. The sun spirit told him, "You possess medicine power for the sun. You could do almost anything with this power. If you like, I can show you a few tricks, but you must promise not to hurt anyone. What I will show you could be very dangerous if you are not careful. You could kill someone!"

Sahlie agreed to be careful because he was very eager to learn about these tricks.

"Here is the sunlight you touched before. Touch it again. Don't be afraid," said the sun spirit. Sahlie cautiously reached for the sunlight and found that, again, it was hard and hot. The sun spirit told him, "Now, use your hand as if it were a knife, and cut through the sunbeam here, and now here."

Sahlie was very surprised to find a length of sunbeam in his hands. To Sahlie, it was a magic wand. The sun spirit said, "This sunbeam is controlled by your mind. It will do whatever you want it to. All you have to do is think it."

Sahlie smiled from ear to ear. The sun spirit told him, "Try this. Gather some dry brush together. Now point the sunbeam at it and think that the end is hot." Suddenly, the leaves ignited into flames. Sahlie laughed out loud. "It is magic!" he thought.

The sun spirit continued to teach Sahlie: "You could cook with this. You could make a hole in the ice when you can go fishing. Or the sunbeam can be cold. Remember, all you have to do is think it cold or hot and it will be. If you make a mistake you could kill someone, so you must be very careful. You can call on me whenever you need me and I will come."

Sahlie was very pleased that he had a sunbeam stick and a spirit teacher that he could call at anytime. The first thing he did was find his best friend. Then Sahlie whispered, "Come with me. I have something to show you!" The two boys ran off together where no one could see them. With pride, Sahlie started a small fire the way the sun spirit had taught him. His friend was very impressed and wanted to try the sunbeam stick himself. Sahlie refused: "No, it's mine and you can never touch it!" To Sahlie it was like a new toy. He played and played with it, honing his skill at using the medicine tool.

But Sahlie was a mischievous boy! He loved to tease the other children. He thought, "I can fool the kids with my sunbeam wand. I know that all I have to do is think that it is cold and it will be, but they don't know that. I could trick them. It will be so funny."

So, the next time Sahlie was playing with the children, he decided to show them the sunbeam stick. The boys and girls were very curious about this stick that looked like sunlight. Then he started a fire with it and they were very surprised.

Sahlie said, "You kids better not bother me or I could cook you alive." Then he waved the sunbeam at them. They all screamed and ran away as fast as they could. Sahlie chased them all around camp and then sat down alone and laughed and laughed. Sahlie was not very popular with the children for his pranks.

The young children ran to their parents and complained that Sahlie was going to "cook them alive" with his sunbeam stick. The parents and Elders were concerned about Sahlie and his behaviour. The Elders asked a group of strong medicine people to have a ceremony to investigate Sahlie and his medicine power. The ceremony took a long time, but finally the group of medicine people were ready to report back to the Elders.

"Sahlie has an unusually large amount of medicine power for the sun. He will be a powerful man when he grows up. In fact, he could be quite dangerous when he is angry. We recommend that you all be very careful with how you treat the boy.".

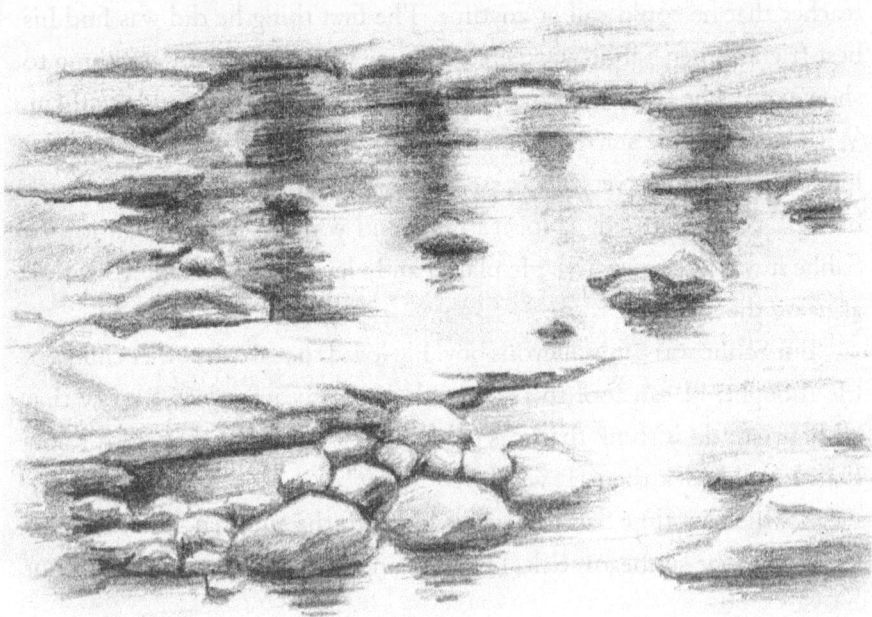

Then the Elders spoke in the gathering place that evening and repeated what the group of medicine people had told them: "Please, remember that Sahlie's gifts could benefit us greatly in the future. Still, he is to be treated with great respect at all times as a precaution. His medicine power could also be very dangerous if used in the wrong way or with anger."

When Sahlie was an adult, the people turned to him for healing when someone was ill. He was good at curing skin problems, and he still had the sunbeam stick. To heal someone he would speak in an unknown language while he rubbed the wand over the sick person. Then they would get better even if they had some kind of internal problem. He was quite famous for this, actually.

AS AN ADULT

Sahlie was a man of action. The people of Sahlie's day were familiar with medicine power because they had opportunities to witness many different medicine people work with their power. Nonetheless, no one had seen anyone like Sahlie.

One day, Sahlie was sitting beside the fire with a group of hunters. Still a show off of his youth, he said, "You know, if I wanted, I could melt your axe and you would have an axe no more."

A hunter spoke up and challenged him: "Talk is cheap. Go ahead!"

Sahlie commanded, "Pass me some lard." He ate the lard, put his hands together, and spoke in a language that no one could understand. Then he picked up the axe in his right hand and held out his left hand palm up. He pushed the head of the axe into the palm of his left hand and the axe began to melt. When he was finished, he was holding a ball of iron in his two hands. Sahlie smiled at the owner of the axe: "See, axe no more. Simple."

The crowd clapped and shook their heads. Soon they were asking him to try it with this old knife and that old file. News spread very fast of Sahlie's performance.

Another time, a large group of Sahlie's people was travelling together. They were really struggling because it was extremely cold. There were no fish lakes, so the group had to count on the caribou for food. Still, they could only find a few.

In the north, when the weather gets too cold, small animals like rabbits, chicken, martin, fox, and mink all disappear into a hole somewhere to stay warm. This made for a desperate situation.

The group had many dogs to feed and feared that they would all starve, dogs and all. Sahlie was with them and thought and thought about how he could help his people. Finally he said, "Maybe I could change the weather for us." Immediately, he began a ceremony. He closed his eyes and spoke in the strange language that he always used to speak to the sun spirit. After a long time he opened his eyes and smiled widely. "Two weeks!" he told them. "The weather will be warm for two weeks. Get ready. We hunt in the morning."

Sure enough, when the group awoke the next morning the sun was shining brightly and the weather was very mild. The group jumped out of their sleeping blankets and set off to hunt. In a short time, they returned with caribou, moose, and many small game fur animals. The people were very grateful to Sahlie and glad that they had such a powerful medicine man among them.

AS AN OLD MAN

Years later, Sahlie went to see the fur trader in Fort Resolution to exchange his furs for some supplies. The manager was a white man who had heard many stories about the famous Sahlie. Still, he did not believe these tales. He told them, "Yeah right. I'll believe that when I see it with my own eyes."

Then when Sahlie actually walked into the Hudson Bay store, he could not resist challenging him right there: "So you're the famous Sahlie who melts iron axes with his bare hands! I've been hoping to meet you some day."

The store was full of people and he was talking loudly, which got everyone's attention. The manager continued, "Sahlie, I'll make you a deal. You see that box with all your supplies. I'll give you the whole box if you can melt iron in front of me."

Sahlie looked up at the store manager with a twinkle in his eye. "I used to be able to do that when I was young but now I'm an old man. I'm losing my power. I can try if you like. Get me a pound of lard and a big file," he told the man.

The store manager retrieved the items and placed them in front of Sahlie. Then Sahlie placed a big chunk of lard in his mouth, opened his left hand, and held the file in his right hand directly above his left hand. He spoke in a strange language and touched the file to his left hand. Immediately it began to melt. When it was melted into his left hand he rolled it into a ball and passed it back to the Hudson Bay store manager. The man was so astonished he could not speak! He just watched as Sahlie casually picked up his box of supplies, turned his back, and walked out of the store smiling widely.

AN EXPLANATION . . .

Sahlie was truly a great medicine-power person. In the time that he lived, there were only four medicine people alive with the strength of medicine power that Sahlie possessed. Sahlie received many, many teachings from the spirit of his medicine power to help him learn how to use his powers.

Sahlie was able to melt iron because he could control the heat of the sun and direct it at objects. When he spoke in the strange language to activate his sun medicine power, he was talking to the sun spirit.

36: The Baby Survives!

ONE SPRING, A GROUP OF MOUNTAIN DENE TRAVELLED DOWN THE river in their moose-skin boats. There were six boats with two families in each boat, including their dogs. Usually, they let the dogs run on shore, but on this river there were too many cut banks and rapids for this practice. They had agreed that they would all wait for each other downstream where the two rivers joined. At that time, the water was low and it was dangerous to travel through the rapids.

The first group arrived at the spot where the two rivers met and set up camp on shore to wait for the others. After four days, the Elders began to worry about the other group. They said, "The water level is very low and that makes the river dangerous. We will send one boat back with five people to paddle up the river to look for them." The five men worked hard paddling all day. They arrived at the rapids by the evening. Just before they got into the canyon there was a wide sandbar near the shore where a small creek came into the river.

They noticed something strange there. An unusual amount of birds and wildlife were sitting on the sandbar. The birds were making a big racket. There were seagulls, ravens, whisky jacks, robins, swans, geese, and other small birds. Then there were also wolverine, fox, bear, and wolves. But as the people neared the sandbar, they all fled.

All that was left was a blanket. When they stopped the boat to investigate, the people were shocked to see a baby in the blanket. They quickly made a fire and tended to the infant. They boiled pounded meat in water and fed him the broth. Then they wrapped him well to keep him warm and headed farther up the river. The broken remains of the moose-skin boat rested along the shore. The area was littered with the belongings of the families who had been riding in the boat. Farther along they found three bodies floating in the water.

With heavy hearts, the men buried their relatives and returned to their people down the river with the unfortunate news. The Elders met and talked among themselves. They questioned, "How could a baby survive all by himself for days on the shore of a river?" They reasoned that the only explanation was that the baby must have medicine power.

They asked four of the strongest medicine men they knew to investigate and find out what they could. The medicine men confirmed that the baby would one day be a very powerful medicine man himself. The Elders found good parents to raise him so that one day he would be able to help the people with his medicine power.

Later, when the baby grew into a teenager, he related how his medicine power saved his life when his family died that day on the river. He said, "I had many visits from the spirits of my medicine power. They told me that they knew when I was in trouble and that they came to my rescue. They told the beaver to come and save me when I fell into the river at the rapids. A beaver swam on each side of me. They held me up until we reached the shore of the sandbar. Then a she-wolf with six pups took me to her den. She nursed me along with her pups.

"A grizzly bear even came with a gift of woodland caribou full of fat. The medicine power spirit knew that my relatives were searching for my family on the river and would soon reach the rapids and find the moose-skin boat. They asked the she wolf to return me to the shore where my relatives could find me. The medicine power spirits of the animals and birds in the area came to visit me on the sandbar. They watched over me and entertained me so that I wouldn't be afraid and cry. They were very noisy. I was quite happy there until my relatives came to rescue me and take care of me."

37: The Story of Batimie

BATIMIE WAS A WELL-KNOWN MEDICINE MAN. HE WAS A GOOD PROVIDER for his family and shared easily with others. He used medicine power to help him hunt, fish, and trap, so he was very successful. In those days there were always many poor people. Batimie would often kill a moose or woodland caribou just to give to other families.

In 1921, there was a big gathering north of Great Bear Lake. At that time, the caribou lived on the Barren lands. They never travelled in the bush like they do today. Dene in the Fort Norman and Colville Lake areas heard about a great herd of caribou and they wanted to see it and hunt. That is why they all travelled to this gathering place on the shore of Great Bear Lake.

It was three hundred miles to the nearest trading post, yet the Dene still travelled all over this vast area hunting for food and trapping fur. You know, Aboriginal people are the kind of people for whom any place in the bush is their home. They are born any place. They die any place. Yet they are happy and rarely worry about anything. When they travel, the whole family sings happy songs to the land. This is how we were in those days.

In the middle of winter, the trappers in the area travelled to the trading posts to sell their furs and buy provisions for the many months ahead. That is where some people said that they planned to head to the Barren lands to see the great caribou herd and make some dry meat. They hoped to catch some white fox, too.

People loaded their toboggans and began the long trek to the Barren lands. Finally they reached a spot about one hundred miles north of Great Bear Lake along the timberline. Soon fifty families populated the area. It was uncommon for so many people to stay in one place because the amount of food needed was so great. Yet, here, it was not a problem because the caribou herd was so large and close.

The people hunted by day and played hand games and danced at night. It was like one long celebration and was a very happy time.

Then something happened that changed all that.

Batimie drove his dogs and sled toward the caribou herd. When he was still a good distance away, he drove a peg in the snowdrift and put on his snow shoes to sneak up closer to get a good shot at a big fat caribou. As he approached he started to run, slipped, and fell. As his rifle hit the ground it went off, shooting him in the head. He screamed and fell to the ground.

Another hunter had witnessed the tragedy and ran to him. Batimie was unconscious on the ground, so the hunter tore his shirt into strips and made bandages for Batimie. It was a grisly sight. Batimie was bleeding badly and his skull was crushed. The hunter was shocked to see Batimie's brain moving where the bone was blown away. He carefully placed the broken pieces of skull back on his head and bandaged him as best as he could.

One look at poor Batimie and people would shake their heads and say, "He is going to die." But still he was alive. They tried to figure out how to transport him the ten miles back to camp. They could not put him on the sled and let the dogs pull him because the snowdrift had made the surface pretty rough and the dogs are fast when they are heading back to camp. The toboggan would bounce up and down and then he would surely die.

Instead, they decided to have four men slowly pull the sled with rope. The rest of the group was loaded down with meat and followed behind the men. Together they reached camp by morning. Amazingly, Batimie was still alive.

Batimie's family gathered in his tent all day. His wife did her best to clean up the sick man. Then they waited. By evening they decided to have a medicine ceremony to help Batimie recovery. Both Kahmosie and Teleway would have separate ceremonies for Batimie.

Kahmosie was first and, after a long ceremony, he announced to the family, "Batimie will not die of this accident. He has some strong medicine powers and they have promised that he will live a long time."

Then Teleway prepared himself for ceremony. He told the relatives that were gathered, "Give me the gun that shot him." He held the gun in both hands, closed his eyes, and began to speak in a strange language. Then he sang. Suddenly he opened his eyes and looked at the people present to address them.

This is what he said: "I have received medicine power for iron and gun powder. You see, in the beginning, the Mother Earth we live on was just a big rock floating in space. First it was part of the sun, but then it broke away to become Mother Earth. I have medicine power for the sun, and because Mother Earth comes from the sun, I also have medicine power for Mother Earth. This gun and powder come from this big rock, so I have the power to control the gun and powder, too."

He held the rifle in both hands, right in the middle, with it pointing crossways. Then he said something in a strange language. Suddenly, the rifle started to shoot. The tent was crowded with people and they started screaming and shouting. It wasn't something that they expected.

Then he tipped the rifle back and rubbed his hand over the wooden handle. The rifle began to smoke until the tent was full of smoke. People were coughing and getting very excited. Teleway stated, "Batimie will not die from this gun." The people were relieved and resumed their busy lives.

Each day, Edward, Batimie's nephew, would go out early in the morning and kill a load of caribou, which is about seven or eight animals. There were many white fox in the area. They were very tame and easy to catch in a trap. So he hunted each day and trapped at the same time.

Edward was a young man and performed most of his work alone. Then, after the day's work and before he went to bed, he would visit his uncle's tent hoping to see Batimie awake and better. However, two weeks after the accident, Batimie was still unconscious.

Edward was getting very concerned. That night he spoke to his uncle, "Please wake up, Uncle. It's been two weeks and you haven't eaten anything." He took the spoon from Batimie's wife and attempted to feed him soup. Then, as the liquid touched Batimie's lips, he swallowed. This was a good sign.

Edward wiped Batimie's face with a wet cloth and slowly fed him soup, spoonful after spoonful. Then Batimie opened his eyes. Edward smiled and said, "Auntie, my uncle opened his eyes. Look!" Then he asked Batimie, "If you can hear me, move your head up and down." Batimie did. Then Edward explained to Batimie what had happened to him and how long he had been unconscious. Batimie tried to talk but it was very difficult for him at first. Later he told them, "All I can remember is hearing a big bang. For one second I thought maybe I would die, but then I remembered the medicine-power spirit that visited me and told me I would live to be an old man."

They were right. Batimie lived to the age of ninety-six.

38: THE STORY OF ADAM

ADAM WAS A MAN FROM FORT GOOD HOPE AND WHAT I LIKE TO call a "small-time medicine person." Adam had a little medicine power, although he liked to boast and talk as if he had a great deal. He was known to use his medicine power to run so fast that he could run down moose and caribou.

Adam often challenged other men to see who was the better hunter or trapper. He also got into a good many fights. At that time, no matter who you were, there was always someone somewhere who had stronger medicine power.

One year a group of people was travelling on the north shore of

Great Bear Lake. They were anxious to hunt beaver and muskrat, so they decided to travel across the lake twenty-six miles to a place known for having these animals.

Adam and his cousin, Karkeyee, chose not to travel with the group but to stay and visit their traps one more time before joining the group. The next day they woke up and set off on their journey. It was early morning and the weather was good. Looking across the land, they could see far away into the distance.

Adam was smiling and seemed very happy. He turned to his cousin and said, "You know, we would make much better time if we ran a little. Do you mind?"

Adam's cousin answered, "Sure, we can run if you want to."

They started off at a nice steady pace. After a while, Adam noticed that little by little Karkeyee was running faster and faster. Soon, Adam was struggling to keep up, but it hurt his pride to show this to Karkeyee because he had been the one asking to run. Adam decided to use his wolf medicine power to help him run like he often did when he hunted caribou and moose.

Still, Karkeyee was running faster than Adam. Frustrated, Adam decided to use his ptarmigan medicine power to fly instead. Karkeyee was disappearing over the lake. Finally, Adam used his loon medicine power but he still couldn't catch Karkeyee.

After a while, Adam noticed smoke on the shore. When he got closer, he saw Karkeyee sitting by the fire cooking meat and grinning from ear to ear. Karkeyee said, "Adam, you must be getting old!"

Adam just shook his head and said in disgust, "For as long as I live, I will never ask you to run again."

Karkeyee thought that was very funny and laughed and laughed and laughed.

AN EXPLANATION

Karkeyee was able to travel far very fast by using mirage medicine power.

Sometimes when you look at something far away it appears to be moving very fast, but it is actually a mirage. Somehow, Karkeyee used this strange phenomenon to help him that day.

39: The Story of Tosoih Taha

TOSOIH TAHA WAS A MAN FROM THE FORT GOOD HOPE AREA. HE WAS well known for his trapping and hunting skills. He was a very generous person, which brought him great respect from everyone. He liked to share the meat and fish he caught, and even the supplies he bought from the trading post. When he brought a big load of provisions back to camp, he would pass out tea, tobacco, sugar, and other things. He never asked for anything in return. He was a wealthy man by the standards of the time.

Whenever a group was travelling to the trading post, you could be sure that Tosoih Taha was with them. He always had furs to trade because he was the best trapper around. Then one year his young daughter was sick with the flu through the best time of trapping season. It was nearing the Christmas season, and, for the first time in his life, he had no furs to trade.

Everyone else, it seemed, was getting ready to go to town to trade their furs and join in the big feast, drum dance, and hand games that were planned. Tosoih Taha wanted to go but had nothing to trade. He felt very disappointed but then decided that with his reputation as a trapper, the fur trader would surely give him some credit this year and allow him to purchase what he needed.

After many days of travel, the group arrived in the town of Fort Good Hope. There were many people about and fur was bringing a very good price. The atmosphere was festive and happy. But the good mood didn't last long for Tosoih Taha. The fur trader refused to allow him credit even for the smallest items.

He was fuming! Without a word, he packed up the few things he had brought with him and took off home with only his dogs and him. He travelled night and day without sleeping until he reached his home camp. His wife was disappointed when she saw him return with an empty sled, but immediately he told her, "I am going hunting right after I get some sleep!"

He set off the next morning with an empty sled yelling, "I'll be right back!" Then a short time later he returned with a sled full of white fox fur. He approached the Elders and women who were left in camp and asked them to dry all the fox pelts. They counted the furs—eighty! No one could trap that many fox in a couple of hours. He told them he would go to town in the morning and they were happy to be able to help such a respected and generous person.

In two short days, Tosoih Taha pulled into Fort Good Hope with a sled full of white fox pelts. When he joined the tea dance he was the loudest and happiest dancer there. People were surprised to see him. A trip that had taken them many days, one way, had taken him only a few days round trip.

AN EXPLANATION . . .

Tosoih Taha was one of the best trappers around because he was gifted with medicine power that helped him to trap. One of the most effective powers that a medicine person can have is mind control. Tosoih Taha was able to catch the animals by controlling their minds and making them do what he wanted. Tosoih Taha used Mother Earth as the floor and some kind of space material as a tunnel. In our language it is called *Yah*. Dene storytellers often tell about a time when someone escaped an enemy by travelling through a hole in the *Yah*.

Tosoih Taha made a tunnel using *Yah* for the fox to run in. He was able to control the fox this way. This time, Tosoih Taha set his traps along that tunnel. Then he sat close by and waited for them to come—all eighty!

40: THE SICK WOMAN IS CURED!

ONE WINTER, AN OLD WOMAN WAS SICK. ALTHOUGH SHE ASKED different medicine people for help, no one was able to cure her. One night, the dogs barked a welcome to two strange dog teams. A group from the Yukon had arrived in camp. The newcomers visited with the people. Then one of the Elders said, "Why don't we ask our guests if any of them could help that poor, sick woman?"

The Elders asked around until one man agreed: "Yes, I'll give it a try."

That evening, they gathered in a tent and had the woman lay on the ground with her feet pointed toward the tent door, an opening in the tent covered by a canvas flap. The man sang in a strange language for a long time. Then he turned to the crowd and said to them, "I cannot do this alone, so I will ask my partner, the Raven, to assist me. Please do not talk while I am performing this ceremony. I will do things so you can see what I am doing. I will also speak in your language so you can hear."

He sang again, and soon the flap of the tent started to move. Suddenly, in jumped a raven, squawking. He settled himself at the head of the sick women. The man sang. The raven squawked. It was quite a racket in the tent. Then they both were quiet. The man spoke to the crowd: "The Raven and I cannot do it alone. We need his wife to help us."

They resumed their singing and squawking and soon the tent flap moved again. Another raven jumped into the tent and settled herself

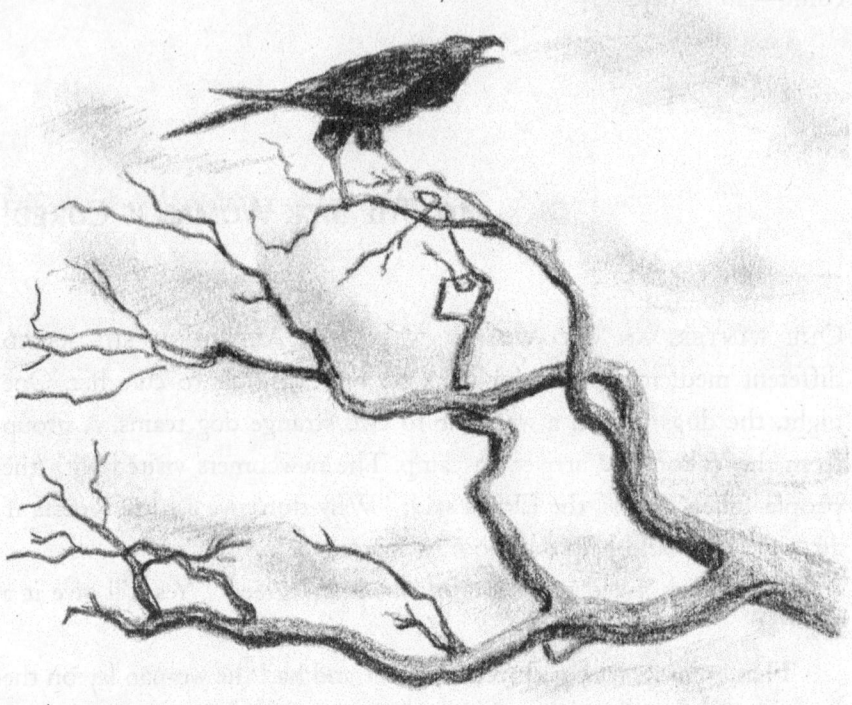

at the feet of the woman. Then all three of them were singing and squawking. The man explained, "Now we will take the sickness out of this poor woman. Make a strong fire. We will have to burn it."

The raven at the head of the woman squawked and squawked. Then he pushed his beak into her stomach and pulled out a large piece of dark meat full of worms. The raven that had been standing at the woman's feet took the piece of meat and dropped it into the fire. Then the raven poked her head out the flap of the tent and flew away. The other followed behind her.

The medicine man told the crowd, "Now this woman will get better!"

And she did.

41: How Medicine Power Stopped Violence in a Family

A strong medicine man was travelling to a trading post. One night he camped with people from another village but planned to leave in the morning to resume his journey. He sat near the fire eating some moose meat when a young woman approached, head down. Silently, she sat near the old man and nervously began to speak: "Grandfather, please listen to what I have to say. I have many problems." Then she began to cry and pushed a beautifully beaded pair of moccasins toward the man.

She said, "These are for you. Please, help me. You see, I have been married to a wicked man for six years already. We have four children together, but my husband is very jealous. He beats me everyday for no reason at all. He accuses me of terrible things, although I have done nothing wrong. If you don't help me, someday he will kill me and then my children will have no mother." With this, the young woman cried very hard.

The old man was sat silently while the woman cried. Finally, he told her, "Tomorrow I leave this place, but I will not forget about you. Your story has touched my heart and I will do what I can to help you."

The young woman whispered, "Thank you."

A year went by until the old man was travelling again in the area. He stopped to visit in the same village. Shortly after he arrived, the young woman approached him again, carrying some beautiful moccasins. She smiled brightly when she handed them to him.

"Thank you" she said. "You have helped change my life. Since that day that I spoke to you last year, my husband is a different man. He has never beaten me again. In fact, I have the best husband in the world. Whatever you did . . . thank you."

AN EXPLANATION...

The Elder and medicine man used mind control to change the young man, and he stayed like that for the rest of his life.

42: THE LEADER OF THE CARIBOU

IN THE NORTH, IN MAY EACH YEAR, WHEN THE SNOW STARTS TO MELT, the caribou travel north. In the past, it was a time when our people worked hard to kill caribou and make dry meat to eat during the summer months.

One year, a boy went caribou hunting with the men. As he travelled he came upon two long lakes and found a well-travelled trail. He thought to himself, "Maybe I should make a fire here and wait for the caribou." But before he could do anything he saw several caribou walk toward the area following the trail. They didn't notice him because there were many willows between him and the trail.

The boy crept closer to hide among the willows where he could get a good shot next time a caribou passed. There he waited.

Caribou have a leader who always travels far ahead of the rest of the herd. Now with Dene people, we have a custom to not shoot the leaders of the caribou. We believe that the leaders are medicine-power caribou and they use their power to take care of the rest of the herd.

The boy knew this because he had been taught well by his father and Elders. He sat waiting for the caribou when the leader of the caribou stopped right in front of him and stared.

When the boy's father and grandfather saw this, they yelled out to the boy, "Don't shoot the leader! Don't shoot the leader! Something bad will happen to you."

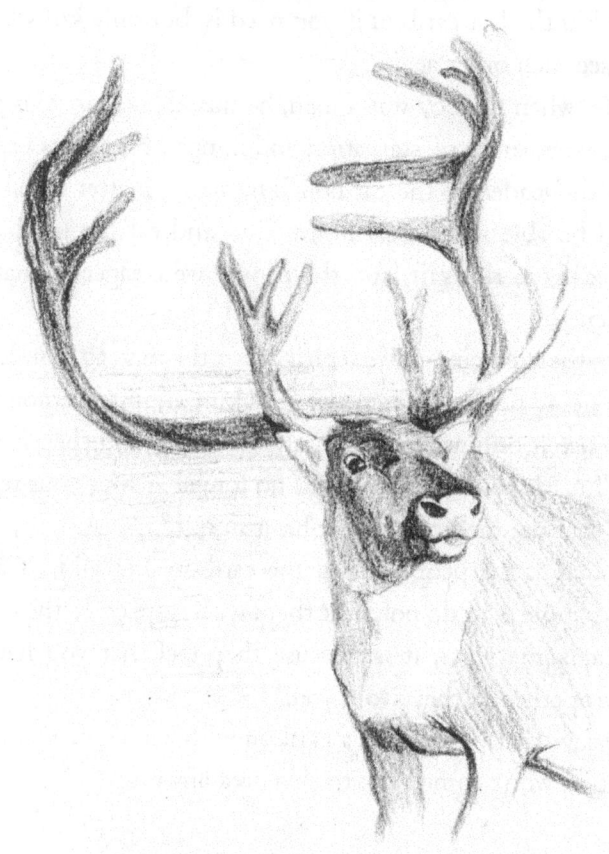

The leader walked right up to the boy. Although it was frightening, the boy was not tempted to shoot the leader. He sat perfectly still, but he was very surprised when the caribou began to talk to him. Suddenly, a smoking pipe sat in front of the boy. "I give you a pipe for you to smoke," the caribou said.

The boy cautiously reached for the pipe and smoked it.

"I will share some of my medicine power with you because I like you," said the caribou. "You are a good person fit for medicine power. Now we will be partners all your life. In the future, if you need me and are hungry, just fill that pipe and think of me. I will come to you right away. You may kill the last caribou if you need it, but only kill what you need. We will see each other again."

Later in life, when the boy was a man, he was able to use this gift to save his people from times of starvation and hunger. He lit his pipe and thought about the leader of the caribou. Then, in a matter of a couple days, he would be able to find caribou to kill and eat for food. Many people benefited from this gift, and the people were eager to make the man their leader.

In this case, the medicine-power spirit asked the man to conserve the use of this medicine power. It seems he gave him a limited amount and wanted him to use it only when absolutely necessary, and then it would last his whole life. He told him, "When I no longer answer your request, you will know that the medicine power has run out."

This man taught the people about the caribou. He said, "Caribou think badly of people who do not treat them with respect. If the caribou don't come near some years, it is because they feel that you have not treated them properly and they avoid you."

Indian law says that if you beat a caribou with a stick or make them suffer, the caribou won't come back to that area any more.

43: WHISKEY JACK MEDICINE

THE PARENTS OF A SMALL BOY WERE VERY ANXIOUS TO HAVE THEIR son receive medicine power. The Elders had told them that, sometimes, if a child sleeps alone in a sacred place, a medicine power spirit will come to him and give him a gift of medicine power. This was exactly what they wanted!

Filled with hope, the small family made the journey to a well-known sacred place. They explained to the boy that he must sleep alone and, if he was lucky, he would receive a gift. They also taught him that medicine power is a secret gift and must never be talked about to anyone, not even them.

Bravely, the young boy slept alone for many nights. Then one night it happened! A vision appeared to the boy. The whiskey jack spirit visited him and said, "You and I are partners. We will be great friends."

When the boy awoke in the morning, he was very excited. He yearned to tell his parents but remembered their teaching him to keep his vision a secret. He could not risk the whiskey jack spirit not coming back. So the boy was silent about it.

As he grew, the whiskey jack spirit visited him many times and taught him how they could work together.

When the boy became an adult and went out hunting, the whiskey jack always flew alongside him. He found that if he followed the bird he would be led to where the moose or caribou were grazing. Soon, he became the best hunter in the country. He shared all that he killed and was a great asset to his people.

This man only received this one item of medicine power, but, still, it was very useful to him throughout his life.

44: THE YEAR OF TWO WINTERS

ONE SPRING, THE SNOW WAS SLOW TO MELT. THEN THE NORTH WIND began to blow and it snowed and snowed. Although the people thought it would soon stop and get warm, it never did. In some places, the snowdrifts were five or six feet deep. The people were astonished, but the spring and then the summer never came. Then winter came again.

The people and animals really suffered that year. It made life very difficult. The snow was so deep that large animals, such as moose, caribou, and sheep, were unable to walk. The hunters found that they could just walk up to the animals and kill them. It was impossible for them to get away.

The Elders talked everyday at the gathering place about the weather. They were very puzzled. They were also worried about the animals. They told the people, "We will have more animals in the future only if we do something to help them now. They will soon starve because of the thick snow."

The people decided to do what they could to save the animals. Instead of spending time hunting, the men spent many days gathering food for animals that were stranded. They piled hay and willows in front of moose and woodland caribou, and even the mountain sheep.

Eventually, the medicine people of the area performed ceremonies to investigate what was behind the strange weather. In this ceremony, they invited many animal spirits to help investigate the reason for the two winters. Some animals reported that there was a medicine power conflict between animals in the north and those in the south—the Alberta area. They said that the southern animals stole the summer away from them. The medicine people asked the squirrel spirit to go into the south and return with the stolen summer.

The next day they had another ceremony. They learned that the squirrel had gone to the south and brought a big bag of warm air back from the summer. Then he poked a hole in it and let it blow the summer back into the land.

Conclusion

I HOPE THAT THIS BOOK HAS GIVEN READERS A BETTER UNDERSTANDING of medicine power. The stories that I have included to illustrate aspects of medicine power are not legends and myths like you may find in other books. Instead, they are real events that happened to real people in and throughout Dene territory. Many of the descendants of the people in the stories live today, here in the North, or in places far away. Some of the events I have actually witnessed myself.

Today, I believe much of the medicine power is being "extinguished," as has been prophesized. They say that we no longer need medicine power to survive and that people have forgotten how to take care of it properly. This is why it is not as prominent as it once was. Many things have changed in just one man's lifetime. That man is me.

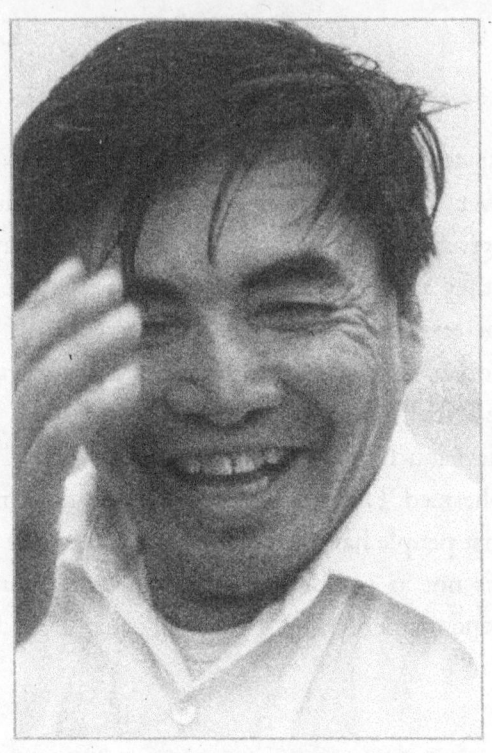

GEORGE BLONDIN is a Dene Elder who was born in 1922 in the Northwest Territories. He has been a wilderness guide, a miner, a trapper, Vice President of the Dene Nation, and, in 1989, was elected Chairman of the Denendeh Elder's Council. He works with the Dene Cultural Institute and writes articles for *News/North*. In 1990, Blondin was the recipient of the annual Ross Charles Award for Native Journalism. He is the author of *When the World was New* and *Yamoria the Lawmaker* and was appointed a member of the Order of Canada in 2003.